The Anthrax Vaccine Debate:
A Medical Review for Commanders

Richard A. Hersack, Col, USAF, MC, CFS

I. Introduction

On 6 February 2000, *60 Minutes* aired an interview of an active duty Air Force major who had refused to receive the vaccine for anthrax.[1] Viewers learned that he faced the potential of a court-martial for refusing to obey orders.[2] The major's refusal is just one aspect of a complex controversy surrounding the Department of Defense's Anthrax Vaccination Immunization Program.[3] Adding to the confusion are a myriad of press releases, communications and opinions from concerned individuals on the internet, Congressional testimony, issues raised by those in the Reserve Components regarding any potential effects on their civilian careers, and numerous internet web sites both supporting and opposing vaccination.

Needless to say the anthrax vaccine debate is extremely complex. It is possible, however, to categorize the issues and concerns with the Anthrax Vaccine Immunization Program as either clinically related or administrative policy related, then address the two categories separately.[4] An important aspect of the clinically related issues is to determine if the anthrax vaccine, Anthrax Vaccine, Adsorbed (AVA), is safe and provides effective protection against the effects of exposure to anthrax spores. What is needed is a clinical assessment based on data in the published, peer-reviewed medical literature and medical textbooks.[5] In addition, it is necessary to assess if credible alternatives to vaccination using Anthrax Vaccine, Adsorbed exist.

If medical personnel determine the vaccine is clinically safe and effective, as documented in the medical literature, then administrative policy-makers may determine if the vaccine should be administered to Department of Defense personnel. The decision to vaccinate Defense Department personnel is a policy decision made by those in the legal chain of command and is based on intelligence estimates and relative risk assessments related to the potential use of anthrax spores in a biological weapon. Clinicians and Service medical corps officers do not set policy. Nor do they have the authority to order vaccination of all personnel.

The intent of this paper is to provide military commanders and supervisors with pertinent clinical facts and information about anthrax and Anthrax Vaccine, Adsorbed in a single source document, written in lay terms, to serve as a working reference for use to educate those within their chain of command. Due to time and space limitations, this paper is not intended to be an exhaustive review.[6] Reviews and discussions of the evidence related to the risk of the use of anthrax as a biological weapon and the policy decision to vaccinate Defense Department personnel are beyond the scope of this paper, which focuses instead on clinical issues related to the vaccine.[7]

The paper will present a brief review of anthrax, including a description of the causative organism and how it causes disease in humans, along with a review of the history of the vaccine and its manufacturer. Next, the paper will provide an overview of the medical literature to address safety, efficacy, side effects, and complications from vaccination, followed by the major points of controversy found in the media, on information world-wide-web sites, and in Congressional testimony. Then, the paper will attempt to bring the controversy into perspective, examining several of the arguments of those opposed to vaccination against anthrax, followed by presenting some conclusions and recommendations. The research methods employed for this paper include a review of the peer-reviewed medical literature, medical textbooks, press releases, and internet world-wide-web sites presenting information and opinions both for and against vaccination.[8]

II. Pathophysiology and Treatment of Human Anthrax Infections

The organism, *Bacillus anthracis,* is a Gram positive (meaning "rod-shaped") bacterium that exists in the soil in dormant spores and can be found throughout the world.[9] The spores are able to exist in the soil for years under the right conditions, such as cool, dry climates, with adequate protection from sunlight.[10] Grazing animals consume the spores that germinate into bacteria inside the animal. The bacteria multiply inside the animal, causing disease, eventually leading to death. After death, the animal's body decomposes, exposing the anthrax bacteria to the air. Oxygen in the air stimulates the bacteria to generate new spores that are released into the environment, either being deposited into the soil or spread by carrion birds and biting insects.[11]

The word "anthrax" comes from the Greek word *anthrakis,* meaning "coal," and refers to the coal-black skin lesions caused when anthrax bacilli infect the skin.[12] Human anthrax has been recognized throughout recorded history. The fifth plague against Egypt recorded in the Book of Exodus in the Bible, and the Torah may have been an outbreak of anthrax.[13] Ancient Greeks, Romans, and Hindus also describe diseases associated with anthrax infection of humans.[14]

In more recent times, certain groups of people such as veterinarians and workers in the goat-hair or wool industries have been identified as having a higher risk of contracting anthrax. During the 1800s, anthrax was a significant agricultural and industrial problem.[15] Indeed, another name for inhalation anthrax is "woolsorters' disease."[16] Exposure to anthrax spores in the work place is effectively controlled through animal vaccination programs, good animal husbandry, vaccinating workers at risk for exposure, and improving working conditions. Such efforts have virtually eliminated anthrax as an occupational hazard in the United Kingdom since 1940.[17] In the United States, human anthrax is extremely rare, with only 224 cases reported over 50 years.[18]

The most recent natural outbreak of human anthrax occurred in Zimbabwe in 1978 and lasted several years. Over 9,700 people became infected and died. Notably, the outbreak was associated with a regional war during which time social services such as animal vaccination programs and medical care broke down, demonstrating the importance of preventive measures programs to control human and animal infection.[19] There has never been a case of human-to-human transmission of anthrax reported, leading most to conclude anthrax is not contagious.[20]

In humans, the anthrax bacillus causes three types of infections: cutaneous, inhalation, and gastrointestinal. Ninety-five percent of human anthrax infections are cutaneous. Spores enter through a break in the skin and germinate to form anthrax bacilli, leading to a localized infection. A vesicle then forms and ruptures to produce the characteristic coal-black lesion. Cutaneous anthrax is easily treated with antibiotics and the lesions heal without scarring. Most patients survive and develop immunity against anthrax.[21] If left untreated, the mortality rate is between 10 and 20 percent.[22]

Inhalation anthrax occurs in five percent of human anthrax infections and is caused when spores enter through the lungs, lodging in the alveoli, the microscopic air sacs where oxygen exchange with the blood occurs. The anthrax spores may reside in the lung alveoli for several weeks before germinating.[23] Macrophages, cells designed to consume foreign bacteria as part of the body's immune system, engulf the spores and then migrate from the lungs to lymph nodes in the chest. Inside the macrophages, the spores germinate, growing into mature anthrax bacilli. The bacilli multiply and eventually erupt from the macrophages, spreading throughout the blood stream.

Initial symptoms of inhalation anthrax signal germination of the spores into mature bacilli and are similar to any common upper respiratory tract infection. Since the symptoms are so non-specific, diagnosis at this point is not possible unless there is reason clinically to suspect anthrax exposure. After a few days, the symptoms subside for a brief period of 12 to 24 hours. This latent period is followed by an explosive period of severe symptoms, shock, and cardiovascular collapse, leading rapidly to death. During this final phase, massive numbers of anthrax bacilli circulate in the blood throughout the body, releasing deadly toxins.

Once initial symptoms develop, nearly 100 percent of all cases of inhalation anthrax are fatal (usually within three days) even with aggressive treatment using antibiotics and supportive intensive medical care. Therefore, if a potential exposure to inhalation anthrax is suspected, treatment must be initiated immediately before any symptoms occur.

Treatment should be continued either until the possibility of anthrax exposure is excluded or no more dormant spores are left in the lungs (usually 60 days).[24]

To develop inhalation anthrax, the subject must inhale a minimum number of spores. The number of spores required to kill at least 50 percent of subjects has been reported to be 8,000 to 10,000 but may range from as few as 2,500 to 5,500.[25] Occupational studies of unvaccinated goat-hair and wool workers demonstrated they inhaled over 500 anthrax spores each day, but they did not develop inhalation anthrax.[26] There have been no cases of inhalation anthrax reported in the United States since 1978 and only 18 cases in the last 80 years.[27]

Without deliberate aerosolization (such as during attack with a biological weapon), it is extremely rare for there to be a sufficient concentration of spores in the inhaled air to cause disease, even if there are large amounts of spores deposited on surfaces or in the soil. Studies indicate that secondary aerosolization typically will not stir up enough spores from contaminated soil or surfaces to achieve sufficient concentrations in inhaled air to cause disease. Therefore, decontamination of large areas and soil is usually not indicated and the presence of residual anthrax spores may not necessarily hinder military operations as some imply.[28]

Gastrointestinal anthrax results from consuming animal products or meat contaminated with anthrax spores. The initial infection occurs either in the mouth and throat or in the intestines. As in inhalation anthrax, macrophages engulf the spores that germinate, forming bacteria that enter the blood stream. The bacteria multiply and release toxins, leading to death in 50 percent of cases. Gastrointestinal anthrax is the rarest form of anthrax infection and has not been reported in the United States.[29]

Rarely, anthrax may also infect the central nervous system, causing hemorrhagic meningitis.[30] This form of anthrax infection does not represent a separate way for anthrax to infect humans. It is actually a complication of cutaneous anthrax, caused by anthrax bacilli spreading through the blood or lymphatic systems to infect the brain and spinal cord.[31] This complication is not frequently seen with inhalation or gastrointestinal anthrax, probably because patients die before meningeal infection by anthrax bacilli occurs. Meningeal anthrax is almost always fatal.

Regardless of the route of infection, death is due to a massive toxic effect from large amounts of toxins produced by overwhelming numbers of anthrax bacilli circulating in the blood. The anthrax bacillus produces three toxins, called protective antigen, edema factor, and lethal factor. The protective antigen binds to the patient's cells, then to either of the other two toxins, forming complexes which penetrate the patient's cells to cause massive cell swelling and rapid cardiovascular collapse.[32] All three toxins work together for anthrax to cause disease. Without the protective antigen, the other two toxins cannot penetrate the cells.

Each anthrax bacillus also forms a protective protein capsule that surrounds the bacillus as it circulates in the blood. The capsule prevents the patient's immune cells from consuming the anthrax bacilli. The anthrax bacillus must be able to produce all three toxins and the protective capsule in order to cause disease in humans.[33] Weakened strains (attenuated) of anthrax bacilli are unable to cause disease in humans because they lack the capability to produce either one or more of the toxins (usually the protective antigen), the protective capsule, or both. These attenuated (weakened) strains are used to produce anthrax vaccines.

The human body normally fights infection two ways: by producing antibodies that circulate in the blood which recognize and attach to foreign proteins, called antigens, and by special cells (such as macrophages) that engulf (called phagocytosis) the bacteria to kill and digest them. Usually these two processes work together. Antibodies bind to antigens on invading bacteria to mark the bacteria. This attracts macrophages to the bacteria so the macrophages may phagocytize them. Antibodies also bind to circulating antigens, produced and released by bacteria into the blood stream, to neutralize their effect.

Anthrax bacilli that are able to cause disease inhibit both parts of the immune process. After coupling with protective antigen, the toxins, edema factor and lethal factor, penetrate into the patient's cells where antibodies in the blood cannot get to them to neutralize their toxic effect. The protective capsule formed by anthrax bacilli in the blood inhibits phagocytosis. As a result, the body's defenses are rendered ineffective.

Understanding these basic concepts is important in order to understand the strategy of treatment regimens and vaccination programs.

The antibiotic of choice for treating anthrax infections is penicillin.[34] For individuals who have an allergy to penicillin, doxycycline is the approved alternative. There are, however, antibiotic resistant strains of anthrax for which neither of these drugs are effective. Ciprofloxacin has been demonstrated in animal studies to be extremely effective against penicillin-resistant anthrax and is recommended by consensus panels as the antibiotic of choice for treating casualties potentially exposed to anthrax spores during an attack.[35] The Food and Drug Administration recently approved ciprofloxacin to treat anthrax in humans.[36]

The treatment strategy for personnel exposed to aerosolized anthrax spores consists of a combination of antibiotics and vaccination. Antibiotics are not effective against toxins and will not prevent the rapid deterioration and death of the patient caused by the toxins. Personnel potentially exposed should receive a vaccination that will stimulate their immune systems to produce antibodies against the toxins (specifically protective antigen) produced by anthrax bacilli, protecting them against the toxins' deadly effects and conferring immunity. But, vaccinating exposed personnel will not kill the anthrax bacilli. Treatment with antibiotics is required to kill the bacilli. This combined therapy of antibiotics and vaccination for inhalation anthrax must begin as soon as exposure to aerosolized anthrax spores is suspected and before any symptoms develop. Once symptoms develop, anthrax spores have already germinated into bacteria that are producing toxins, and death will most likely occur in spite of treatment.[37]

III. Anthrax Vaccine, Adsorbed (AVA)

Anthrax Vaccine, Adsorbed is the Food and Drug Administration's approved and licensed vaccine for use to immunize humans against anthrax infection. The strain of anthrax bacteria used to make Anthrax Vaccine, Adsorbed lacks the ability to make the protective capsule (cannot prevent the body's defensive macrophages from phagocytizing the bacteria) and is unable to produce disease in humans. There are no live bacteria and no intact cells in the vaccine, so it is impossible to get infected with anthrax from the vaccine. The vaccine consists of protective antigen isolated from these attenuated (unable to produce disease) anthrax bacteria.[38] Protective antigen has been shown to be the essential antigen for provoking the immune response against anthrax in both animals and humans. Every anthrax vaccine developed that has been demonstrated as effective in immunizing test subjects against anthrax involves the use of protective antigen as the primary agent to trigger the immune response.[39] After injection, the vaccine stimulates the individual's immune system to produce antibodies against protective antigen, which protect the individual from future infections by anthrax bacilli. After vaccination, it takes the individual some time to develop enough immunity to confer protection and one dose may or may not be fully protective.[40] Therefore, a non-immunized person exposed to aerosolized anthrax spores, in addition to immediate vaccination with the anthrax vaccine, requires treatment with antibiotics to prevent disease.

The current dosage schedule approved by the Food and Drug Administration (FDA) for Anthrax Vaccine, Adsorbed is three injections 2 weeks apart followed by three more injections 6 months apart. After the completed course, an annual booster is required to maintain immunity. Animal and human studies suggest that Anthrax Vaccine, Adsorbed may confer immunity with fewer doses. But, since the vaccine is currently licensed with the six-dose regimen, this regimen should be followed until clinical studies confirm adequate protection could be achieved with fewer doses.

Formaldehyde (up to 0.02 percent) is used as a stabilizer in Anthrax Vaccine, Adsorbed and benzethonium chloride (0.0025 percent) as a preservative.[41] The Food and Drug Administration has approved the use of formaldehyde in trace amounts as a preservative.[42] The use of formaldehyde as a preservative is actually quite common and has been done for the past 40 years. For example, tetanus toxoid, given to all school children in the United States, contains trace amounts of formaldehyde, yet it has been used safely for decades to induce immunity in millions of people by stimulating the production of antibodies against tetanus.[43]

Anthrax Vaccine, Adsorbed does not contain, nor has it ever contained, squalene as an additive. Squalene is a substance sometimes used to increase the potency of certain vaccines.[44] Squalene occurs naturally in humans and is a precursor in the synthesis of cholesterol.[45] Squalene is also found in large amounts in deep-sea shark liver. There are currently several health food supplemental products on the market containing squalene. Proponents claim squalene improves the delivery of oxygen to cells and facilitates the clearance of metabolic toxins.[46]

Recent reports have stated that newly developed tests have detected trace amounts of squalene in Anthrax Vaccine, Adsorbed and other commonly used vaccines.[47] Previous tests were only able to detect the presence of squalene in parts per million, but the newer, more sensitive tests are able to measure the presence of squalene down to the parts per billion. The concentration of squalene detected in the anthrax vaccine, diphtheria vaccine, and tetanus toxoid, using the newer tests, is about ten parts per billion. The normal concentration of squalene circulating in human blood is many times higher, about 250 parts per billion, suggesting the presence of trace amounts of squalene in the anthrax vaccine is not clinically significant. The presence of trace amounts of squalene in the anthrax vaccine and in the other vaccines may be a normal bi-product of the production process.[48]

There have been articles in the press attempting to draw a connection between the use of Anthrax Vaccine, Adsorbed and Gulf War Syndrome, claiming the agent causing Gulf War Syndrome is squalene. These press reports claim veterans suffering from Gulf War Syndrome have antibodies to squalene in their blood that they got from Anthrax Vaccine, Adsorbed.[49] Others have gone so far as to charge the Defense Department may have secretly added squalene to lots of the vaccine used for inoculation of troops to increase its efficacy. They claim, without presenting any evidence, that Anthrax Vaccine, Adsorbed vial labels may have been altered and that lack of documentation in personal shot records suggests a cover-up.[50]

IV. History of Production

Merck, Sharp & Dohme developed the first anthrax vaccine for use in humans during the 1950s to protect workers routinely exposed to anthrax spores.[51] Clinical trials performed in the late 1950s and published in 1962 demonstrated that the vaccine was effective in preventing cutaneous anthrax.[52] Later, the Department of Defense approached the state of Michigan to manufacture anthrax vaccine for Defense Department personnel. The Defense Department chose the state of Michigan because there was little profit potential to motivate private industry to manufacture a vaccine that would not be used in the general public, and Michigan had extensive experience manufacturing other vaccines such as rabies vaccine.

The Michigan Biological Products Institute began to produce Anthrax Vaccine, Adsorbed for the Defense Department. Anthrax Vaccine, Adsorbed is essentially the same vaccine as initially produced by Merck, Sharp & Dohme except that Anthrax Vaccine, Adsorbed is more potent and more pure, due to some minor differences in production technique.[53] In 1970, the National Institute of Health's Division of Biologics Standards licensed Anthrax Vaccine, Adsorbed, then transferred the license, along with oversight and regulatory authority, to the Food and Drug Administration in 1972.[54] Licensing was based on data collected during studies using the older anthrax vaccine and Anthrax Vaccine, Adsorbed to protect workers at risk for infection. The study using the older, less potent vaccine (published in 1962) measured the older vaccine's effectiveness to protect wool mill workers at risk for both cutaneous and inhalation anthrax. The Centers for Disease Control and Prevention collected data over a 10-year period, after 1960, using Anthrax Vaccine, Adsorbed to measure how effectively it prevented cutaneous anthrax in workers at risk for infection. Of note, the licensing procedures also cited the demonstrated low risk of serious side effects.[55]

As tensions in the Persian Gulf mounted in early 1990, the Defense Department asked Michigan Biological Products Institute to dramatically increase the production rate of Anthrax Vaccine, Adsorbed.[56] Michigan Biological Products Institute informed the Defense Department it would not be able to meet production expectations with the facilities it possessed at that time. Michigan Biological Products Institute then worked out a plan with the Defense Department to upgrade their production facilities with Defense Department funding and presented the plan to the Food and Drug Administration in 1995. The Food and Drug Administration approved the facility upgrade plans.

Between 1995 and 1997, the Food and Drug Administration performed several inspections of Michigan Biological Products Institute's facilities used to produced rabies vaccine and plasma derivative products. During these inspections, the Food and Drug Administration found numerous discrepancies with policies and procedures, record keeping, analytical laboratories, quality control practices, raw materials handling, filling and packaging, and storage, warehousing, and distribution.[57] It must be noted that none of these production facilities, nor any of the Food and Drug Administration's findings, involved the production, safety, or quality of Anthrax Vaccine, Adsorbed. In March 1997, the Food and Drug Administration sent Michigan Biological Products Institute a letter indicating the they would begin procedures to revoke Michigan Biological Products Institute's license due to lack of adequate progress to address the discrepancies noted during the inspections of the facilities used to produce rabies vaccine and plasma derivative products.

In the meantime, Michigan Biological Products Institute had applied to the Food and Drug Administration to upgrade its Anthrax Vaccine, Adsorbed production facilities to meet the increased demand for vaccine resulting from the Defense Department's Anthrax Vaccine Immunization Program. The Food and Drug Administration approved the planned upgrade and, in January 1998, Michigan Biological Products Institute voluntarily stopped production of Anthrax Vaccine, Adsorbed in order to begin the Food and Drug Administration-approved renovations to the production facilities. It is important to note that the stoppage of production of the Anthrax Vaccine, Adsorbed is completely unrelated to the discrepancies noted during the Food and Drug Administration inspections of rabies vaccine and plasma derivative products production facilities and is completely unrelated to their letter of intent to revoke Michigan Biological Products Institute's license.

In 1997, Secretary of Defense Cohen made the decision to implement the Anthrax Vaccine Immunization Program (AVIP) to vaccinate all military personnel using lots of Anthrax Vaccine, Adsorbed already on hand. Since supplies of the vaccine were limited, the immunization program was divided into three phases. Completion depended on the production and release to the Department of Defense of additional lots of vaccine after the production facilities were upgraded. Only the first phase has been implemented, meaning only personnel at risk for exposure to inhalation anthrax in high risk areas (i.e., Korea and the Persian Gulf) will be vaccinated.

Part of the Secretary's directive was that each lot of vaccine would be completely re-tested (referred to as "supplemental testing") using Food and Drug Administration testing procedures to reconfirm potency, safety, purity, and sterility. Each lot had to pass supplemental testing before it would be administered to Defense Department personnel. The lots undergoing supplemental testing had already passed Food and Drug Administration certification, been released by them for sale, and purchased by the Defense Department.

Eight lots have undergone this supplemental testing for potency and were released before a problem with the potency test itself was discovered in the Fall of 1998.[58] Since then, the potency testing difficulties have been corrected and the test is now working according to specifications.[59] But, the Food and Drug Administration will not release any additional lots until it is satisfied with the quality of the vaccine and has approved necessary potency test amendments implemented to correct the earlier potency testing problems.[60]

In September 1998, the state of Michigan sold the Michigan Biological Products Institute facilities with the licensing rights to BioPort as part of an effort to privatize government programs and cut costs.[61] In late 1999, BioPort completed the renovations and applied to the Food and Drug Administration for inspection and certification of the new production facilities.[62] But BioPort continues to have problems with its renovated facility and still has not received Food and Drug Administration certification.[63]

In the meantime, BioPort has started producing new lots of anthrax vaccine.[64] It is important to note that the new lots produced by BioPort have not been certified or released for sale by the Food and Drug Administration, have not been purchased by the Defense Department, and have not been administered to anyone. Furthermore, the Defense Department will not purchase these lots to begin Phase Two of the Anthrax Vaccine Immunization Program until the BioPort facility passes Food and Drug Administration inspection and they have tested, certified, and released the new lots for distribution.[65]

BioPort has a total of 32 lots of Anthrax Vaccine, Adsorbed in storage for the Defense Department, produced by the Michigan Biological Products Institute division before the production facilities were shut down for renovations. In February 1998, the Food and Drug Administration inspected these lots of vaccine and Michigan Biological Products Institute voluntarily quarantined 10 lots mentioned in the Food and Drug Administration report. The Defense Department has not used these lots for the immunization program. These lots will remain quarantined until testing confirms adequate sterility, potency, and quality to the Food and Drug Administration's satisfaction.[66] In addition, one other lot was permanently quarantined due to questions regarding sterility and will not be used. Furthermore, 14 lots were tested at random and found not to contain any squalene.[67]

Most recently, the rate of vaccination of Defense Department personnel under the Anthrax Vaccine Immunization Program has been reduced due to the dwindling supply of vaccine. As of May 2000, 17 lots of vaccine have passed Food and Drug Administration certification tests and passed re-certification tests as ordered by the Secretary of Defense.[68] Defense Department officials have pointed out on numerous occasions in the media and in sworn testimony that only these 17 lots have been used for the immunization program.

Defense Department officials had hoped that BioPort would have obtained Food and Drug Administration approval and new lots tested and released by the Food and Drug Administration by now.[69] Due to ongoing problems with BioPort obtaining certification (the Food and Drug Administration has identified 30 deficiencies that need to be rectified before it grants certification), no new lots are available for the immunization program, forcing the slowdown in the program. In addition, some members of Congress who are dissatisfied with BioPort's situation are beginning to urge the Defense Department to consider designing a

Government Owned, Contractor Operated (GOCO) vaccine production facility.[70]

In summary, it should be noted that Anthrax Vaccine, Adsorbed is a Food and Drug Administration licensed, non-experimental vaccine. Anthrax Vaccine, Adsorbed is more potent and purer than, but otherwise identical to, the earlier version of the vaccine produced in the 1950s by Merck, Sharp & Dohme. Michigan Biological Products Institute voluntarily stopped production of Anthrax Vaccine, Adsorbed in order to upgrade the vaccine production facilities, not due to the results of any Food and Drug Administration inspections. Michigan Biological Products Institute then sold its Anthrax Vaccine, Adsorbed production facilities to BioPort.

The lots currently in use for the Anthrax Vaccine Immunization Program were produced before the renovations began, tested and certified by the Food and Drug Administration for release and distribution, and re-tested by the Defense Department before administration. No lots produced by BioPort since it purchased and renovated the Michigan Biological Products Institute production facilities have been used by the Defense Department to vaccinate its personnel. The Defense Department-mandated supplemental testing, BioPort's voluntary quarantine of lots previously released by the Food and Drug Administration, and the modifications implemented to improve the quality of testing for potency demonstrate the intense level of interagency scrutiny that exists to ensure the Defense Department's Anthrax Vaccine Immunization Program attains the highest possible levels of safety for its personnel.

V. Efficacy

A controlled study using the original anthrax vaccine produced by Merck, Sharp & Dohme and supplied by the U.S. Army Chemical Corps was published by Brachman, et al., in 1962.[71] The study looked at how effectively the vaccine prevented anthrax in a population of wool mill workers considered to be at risk for contracting anthrax. Historically, about one percent of these workers contracted cutaneous anthrax annually. To do the study, volunteers were divided into two groups—one group received the vaccine and the other received a placebo (an inactive substance used as a control that looks like the vaccine, but is harmless and has no biological effect). The vaccination schedule used in the study matches the current Food and Drug Administration approved schedule for vaccinations using Anthrax Vaccine, Adsorbed. The rate of occurrence of anthrax in the vaccinated group was compared to the rate of occurrence in the group that received the placebo and all other workers not participating in the study.

During the study period there were 26 cases of anthrax. One case of cutaneous anthrax appeared in a fully vaccinated individual. Twenty-three cases of anthrax appeared in unvaccinated workers and two in partially vaccinated (meaning they did not complete the series of immunizations) workers. No cases of inhalation anthrax occurred in vaccinated or partially vaccinated workers, although five cases of inhalation anthrax occurred in unvaccinated workers during the study period. Four of these cases were fatal. The frequency of occurrence of inhalation anthrax was not sufficient to determine any statistical significance for how effective the vaccine was in preventing inhalation anthrax.[72]

As already pointed out, the vaccine used in the Brachman study was also a protective antigen vaccine similar to Anthrax Vaccine, Adsorbed, but less potent and less pure (it contained more cell fragments). Since the mechanism to produce immunity is the same for both vaccines, Brachman's study results are relevant when discussing the issue of efficacy of Anthrax Vaccine, Adsorbed. In addition, other surveillance studies using Anthrax Vaccine, Adsorbed completed since the publication of Brachman's study confirm the vaccine's efficacy in preventing anthrax in humans.[73]

Between 1962 and 1974, the Centers for Disease Control and Prevention (CDC) collected data measuring the occurrence of anthrax in workers at risk for infection who had been vaccinated with Anthrax Vaccine, Adsorbed versus non-immunized workers. The study also tracked any adverse reactions to the vaccine.[74] During this period, an additional 27 cases of cutaneous anthrax were identified, three in partially immunized workers who had only received one or two doses. There were no cases of anthrax in the fully immunized workers.[75] A total of 7,000 workers received more than 16,000 doses of Anthrax Vaccine, Adsorbed.[76] The efficacy data from the Brachman study, using the original protective antigen vaccine, and the Centers for Disease Control and Prevention study, using Anthrax Vaccine, Adsorbed, were eventually used during the licensing procedures for Anthrax Vaccine, Adsorbed.[77]

Between 1974 and 1989, it is estimated that an additional 68,000 doses of Anthrax Vaccine, Adsorbed were administered to at risk individuals.[78] There were no cases of cutaneous anthrax in vaccinated individuals although there continued to be reported cases of cutaneous anthrax in unvaccinated people at risk. In addition, the rate of adverse side effects remained low, comparable to rates cited in the Food and Drug Administration-required package insert that accompanies each vial of Anthrax Vaccine, Adsorbed.[79] Due to the increasing rarity of anthrax infections, the fact that workers at risk for exposure to anthrax spores are immunized, and improvements in working conditions, any additional field studies of anthrax vaccine are unlikely.[80] In conclusion, the clinical data collected over several decades indicate that Anthrax Vaccine, Adsorbed is very effective in preventing cutaneous anthrax and, potentially, inhalation anthrax in humans.[81]

Fortunately, inhalation anthrax in humans is very rare even among unvaccinated workers routinely exposed to anthrax spores. Improvements in the work place plus use of Anthrax Vaccine, Adsorbed in workers at risk for exposure to anthrax spores essentially eliminated the occurrence of inhalation anthrax.[82] But, the rareness of this disease also means it is not possible to collect enough data in humans to determine if Anthrax Vaccine, Adsorbed would prevent inhalation anthrax in humans. In order to do a study in humans, one would have to take volunteers, divide them into two groups, vaccinate one group with Anthrax Vaccine, Adsorbed, the other with a placebo. Then the experiment would have to expose both groups to lethal doses of aerosolized anthrax spores, and track how many in each group contract the disease. Obviously, any such study would be unethical, illegal, and should not take place.

Numerous animal studies have been performed to measure the effectiveness of Anthrax Vaccine, Adsorbed to prevent inhalation anthrax. Granted, there is always a possibility that results in one species of animals cannot be assumed to represent potential results in another species. For example, animal studies suggest that some species are more difficult to immunize against anthrax infections, using Anthrax Vaccine, Adsorbed, than others. In guinea pigs, Anthrax Vaccine, Adsorbed seems to confer variable protection against certain strains of anthrax, suggesting possible species-dependent differences in the guinea pig's immune system. Guinea pigs seem especially sensitive to one particular strain of anthrax, called the Ames strain, even after they are fully immunized with Anthrax Vaccine, Adsorbed.

On the other hand, Anthrax Vaccine, Adsorbed confers excellent protection in rabbits and non-human primates against the Ames strain, providing near 100 percent protection even after as few as two inoculations, including situations where they are exposed to several times the lethal dose of anthrax spores. Moreover, inhalation anthrax infections in non-human primates closely resemble inhalation anthrax infections in humans.[83] Based on the animal studies results and the absence of cutaneous and inhalation anthrax in fully immunized individuals exposed to anthrax spores, it is reasonable to conclude that Anthrax Vaccine, Adsorbed prevents inhalation anthrax in humans.[84]

VI. Side Effects and Safety

The side effects and adverse reactions recognized as caused by Anthrax Vaccine, Adsorbed tends to be grouped into four main categories: mild local reactions, moderate local reactions, severe local reactions, and systemic reactions. Mild local reactions are defined by tenderness and redness in an area less than 1 to 2 cm in diameter and occur about 30 percent of the time. Moderate local reactions are identified by an area of response greater than 5 cm in diameter and occur about 4 percent of the time. Severe local reactions are characterized by extensive swelling (edema) of the arm and forearm in which the vaccine was administered. These occur less frequently than moderate reactions. In general, the rate of local reactions is about twice as high in women than men.[85] Systemic reactions are characterized by fever, chills, nausea, and body aches and occurs in less than 0.2 percent of vaccinations.[86] Allergic reactions are even less common, being reported in only one per 100,000 doses.[87]

Normally it takes three doses of Anthrax Vaccine, Adsorbed before an individual begins to develop an immune response and seem to correlate with the observation that reactions to subsequent doses of Anthrax Vaccine, Adsorbed tend to be stronger.[88] Individuals who have had cutaneous anthrax or who have severe local or systemic reactions to the vaccine are not to receive Anthrax Vaccine, Adsorbed.[89] In a study conducted from 1962 to 1974, the Centers for Disease Control and Prevention tracked the occurrence rates of reactions during the administration of more than 16,000 doses of Anthrax Vaccine, Adsorbed to over 7,000 individuals. The results of this study are the rates reported on the informational package insert accompanying each vial of Anthrax Vaccine, Adsorbed as required by the Food and Drug Administration.[90]

Since Anthrax Vaccine, Adsorbed was licensed in 1970, there have been numerous reviews documenting the occurrence of side effects attributable to Anthrax Vaccine, Adsorbed. An independent civilian advisory panel met in 1985 to review the results of the 1962 to 1974 Centers for Disease Control and Prevention study.[91] The panel reported that only a few systemic side effects had occurred which all resolved. Local reactions were typically mild and also resolved.[92] From 1974 to 1989, over 68,000 doses of vaccine were administered to persons considered at risk for contracting anthrax (such as goat-hair workers, laboratory personnel, livestock handlers, and veterinarians). Yet, after more than 30 years of use, no long-term side effects have been reported in association with Anthrax Vaccine, Adsorbed.[93]

Since 1973, the U.S. Army Medical Research Institute of Infectious Diseases (USAMRIID) at Fort Detrick, Maryland, has actively followed 1,590 workers who have received more than 10,000 doses of Anthrax Vaccine, Adsorbed, again with no reported long-term or chronic side effects. Only 4 percent reported local reactions and only 0.5 percent had any type of systemic reactions. All reactions resolved without any lost work time.[94] Another study conducted by the Canadian Armed Forces reported that in 547 individuals who received Anthrax Vaccine, Adsorbed, rates of reaction were less than the rates listed on the Anthrax Vaccine, Adsorbed package insert. There were no long-term effects except for one individual who reported a persistent nodule at the injection site.[95]

In addition to the Centers for Disease Control and Prevention study, the USAMRIID study, and the Canadian study, there are three other separate studies on Anthrax Vaccine, Adsorbed, examining the rate of occurrence of adverse reactions. In 1997, Pittman reported on 508 subjects who were actively followed after they received Anthrax Vaccine, Adsorbed. Local reaction rates were roughly the same as reported by other studies. But Pittman noted a much higher rate of systemic reactions. Twenty-nine percent were classified as mild and 14 percent were classified as moderate to severe. Another study, conducted at Tripler Army Medical Center in Hawaii, reported a rate of mild systemic effects of 43 percent and moderate to severe in 5 percent out of a total of 536 individuals vaccinated. Both studies are significant in that they report moderate to severe systemic reactions much higher than the 0.05 percent to 0.2 percent usually reported. And they differentiate between mild and moderate to severe systemic reactions.[96]

The third study is an ongoing Department of Defense study which reported in May of 1999 that out of 223,000 individuals vaccinated, 42 experienced adverse side effects which were reported to the Food and Drug Administration and the Centers for Disease Control and Prevention. Of these, seven either missed more than one day of work or required hospitalization. None of these studies note any long-term or chronic adverse effects attributable to Anthrax Vaccine, Adsorbed and none question the safety of the vaccine in their conclusions.[97] In addition, there have been no cases of anaphylactic reactions (severe, potentially life threatening, systemic allergic reactions) reported due to Anthrax Vaccine, Adsorbed administration.[98]

There have been multiple review panels, including panels hosted by the Food and Drug Administration, the Centers for Disease Control and Prevention, the World Health Organization, and the Armed Forces Epidemiological Board. Most recently, a civilian panel of 21 experts from several major medical and research centers led by Dr. Thomas V. Inglesby convened to assess the risk that anthrax could be used as a biological weapon agent. The panel also developed a consensus on the care and management of victims of an anthrax biological weapon attack and examined the safety and efficacy of Anthrax Vaccine, Adsorbed. The panel's results were published in May 1999 in the *Journal of the American Medical Association.*[99]

The panel concluded that the likelihood that anthrax could be used in a terrorist attack is high. The panel also reported that its investigation of the clinical data on the use of Anthrax Vaccine, Adsorbed showed no serious adverse effects have been causally related to the vaccine, and they reached a consensus for recommending treatment protocols to care for anthrax victims. The panelists recommended that new research should be devoted to developing a next-generation anthrax vaccine that requires fewer doses to immunize humans. Their findings correlate with the findings of numerous other review panels examining the medical literature published on Anthrax Vaccine, Adsorbed, which confirm the clinical safety and the efficacy of the vaccine in humans.[100]

In 1990, the Food and Drug Administration and Centers for Disease Control and Prevention launched the Vaccine Adverse Events Reporting System. This is a passive reporting system, meaning success depends on medical personnel, patients, and families taking the initiative to file reports. As of 23 August 2000, 1,859,666 doses of Anthrax Vaccine, Adsorbed have been administered to 463,027 personnel with 945 reports submitted to the Vaccine Adverse Events Reporting System. Of these reports, 492 were determined to be actually due to Anthrax Vaccine, Adsorbed -- 374 were less than serious, 111 reported a loss of more than 24 hours of duty, and 7 were hospitalized for allergic inflammatory reactions at the injection site. All symptoms resolved and there were no permanent side effects.[101]

In addition to the Food and Drug Administration reviews of the Vaccine Adverse Events Reporting System data, the Defense Department convened the Anthrax Vaccine Executive Committee composed of non-government medical experts. This committee meets periodically to review the Vaccine Adverse Events Reporting System reports.[102] Since its first meeting in 1990, the committee has not identified any unexpected patterns of adverse events among the reports submitted to the Vaccine Adverse Events Reporting System.[103] The committee continues to meet every six weeks to review data reported on the vaccine.[104]

To date, the Anthrax Vaccine Executive Committee has concluded it is not possible to attribute to Anthrax Vaccine, Adsorbed all the symptoms reported to the Vaccine Adverse Events Reporting System. But, for the sake of argument, if one assumes that all the reports could be linked causally to the vaccine, the rate of adverse reactions, including serious or severe ones, is still less than 0.03 percent. This is below the rate of 0.05 percent reported by other studies and well below the rate of 0.2 percent listed in the Anthrax Vaccine, Adsorbed product information package insert. By way of comparison, the hepatitis B vaccine, required for all health care workers, has a systemic reaction rate five times greater than that observed due to Anthrax Vaccine, Adsorbed.[105] Based on the Vaccine Adverse Events Reporting System data, the Food and Drug Administration has concluded that it has no concerns about the safety of Anthrax Vaccine, Adsorbed and "continues to view the anthrax vaccine as safe and effective for individuals at risk of exposure to anthrax."[106]

In all there have been at least 13 studies conducted in humans assessing the safety of Anthrax Vaccine, Adsorbed or its precursor protective antigen vaccine, including those discussed in this paper, covering almost 50 years of clinical experience.[107] The clinical evidence accumulated is consistent from study to study and demonstrates that Anthrax Vaccine, Adsorbed is safe and effective. This vaccine quite possibly has undergone more scrutiny than any other vaccine developed for human use, yet it continues to find endorsement in medical textbooks, in the medical peer-reviewed literature, and in sworn testimony given before Congressional panels as a safe and reliable vaccine against human anthrax infections.[108]

VII. The Threat of Anthrax as a Biological Weapon, and Policy Decisions

As stated in the introduction, the main purpose of this paper is to provide an overview of the use of Anthrax Vaccine, Adsorbed from a clinical perspective to determine if the vaccine is clinically safe and effective. The decision to vaccinate all Defense Department personnel against anthrax is a policy decision that is based on available intelligence estimates that an attack against U.S. personnel may occur using anthrax as a biological agent. A review of all the evidence used to make that decision is beyond the scope of this paper. Suffice it to say, there is a clear consensus in the literature and the media among senior Defense Department officials and policy-makers that the threat posed by the potential use of anthrax against U.S. military personnel is real and significant.[109]

Several reports and testimonies document how easy it is to acquire, grow, and weaponize anthrax spores.[110] Evidence confirms the existence of active biological programs in the former Soviet Union, Iraq, and at least five other nations involving ongoing efforts to develop and stockpile anthrax weapons.[111] In addition, various U.S. agencies receive terrorist threats against U.S. interests each day.[112] In light of this evidence, many feel the U.S. is under-prepared to deter or respond to a biological attack.[113] But even though the U.S. may be under-prepared, many are opposed to the use of Anthrax Vaccine, Adsorbed to protect U.S. military personnel from the biological agent most likely to be used in an attack. Recently, a bill has been introduced in Congress calling for suspension of the Defense Department Anthrax Vaccine Immunization Program.[114]

Many believe that the most likely place U.S. troops would face attack from an anthrax weapon is on the battlefield in an open conflict where the mortality rate could be as high as 80 percent.[115] One pilot refusing to take Anthrax Vaccine, Adsorbed stated in an interview that if a war occurs, he will submit to vaccination against anthrax.[116] But, other staff studies conclude the least likely use of anthrax as a weapon would be overtly on the battlefield during a war.[117] These argue that it is much more likely that a terrorist group or covert operator would use an anthrax-based biological weapon as a weapon of stealth.[118]

Currently, the U.S. does not possess the capability to detect and warn of a small-scale biological attack at the time it occurs. Current detection systems do not provide comprehensive real-time detection and warning. Furthermore, if the agent is not released upwind of a detection unit, the unit may not detect the agent at all. Indeed, the first indication that an attack using anthrax has occurred may be the outbreak of symptoms.[119] Protective masks issued by the military do provide passive protection. But, to be effective, protective masks must be worn at the time of attack. Since detection and early warning are not possible, protective masks would have to be worn at all times to provide effective protection from anthrax, and because it takes time for an individual to develop an immune response after inoculation with Anthrax Vaccine, Adsorbed, immunization at the time an attack using anthrax as a weapon is believed to be imminent will not provide any protection.[120] Therefore, the best, and most practical, real-time protection currently available against an anthrax weapon attack is prior vaccination.

Vaccination of all military personnel against anthrax could provide a powerful deterrent against any attack by an adversary using biological agents. As already pointed out, anthrax is the cheapest and most easily weaponized agent of all potential biological agents. It is also potentially the most effective, making it the most likely biological agent an adversary would select to attack our forces. If our forces are protected against anthrax, a potential adversary probably will not have an alternative biological agent to employ as a weapon. Furthermore, fully immunizing our military personnel should deter any attack using anthrax since the effects of such an attack would likely be small and not worth the risk and costs of triggering a retaliation against the attacker by the United States.

No vaccine is totally risk-free and complications from vaccination will occur. All vaccines have potential adverse reactions that could be severe. Vaccination programs should only be undertaken when the risk of contracting a disease, with its associated complications, outweigh the risks associated with vaccination. In other words, the decision to vaccinate should be based on risks versus benefits analysis, weighing the potential risk that biological attacks with anthrax weapons could occur against the potential risks of reactions to the vaccine. The risk that an anthrax weapon could be used to attack U.S. military personnel is significant, and the disease caused by the weapon, inhalation anthrax, is highly lethal. By contrast, the clinical evidence we have today shows that Anthrax Vaccine, Adsorbed is at least as safe as any other vaccine currently in use today and its efficacy in preventing anthrax disease in persons exposed to aerosolized anthrax spores is high. Therefore, based on this risk-benefit analysis, the policy decision to implement the Anthrax Vaccine Immunization Program is reasonable.

VIII. Arguments Against Anthrax Vaccine, Adsorbed

A number of informational world-wide-web sites exist opposing the Defense Department's Anthrax Vaccine Immunization Program to vaccinate military personnel against anthrax using Anthrax Vaccine, Adsorbed. One of the most comprehensive is entitled "Anthrax Vaccine Links and Information" and provides an extensive list of links to other related sites. Included are links to sites with copies of Congressional testimony, General Accounting Office reports, summaries of the symptoms reported by personnel at Dover Air Force Base, Delaware, who received Anthrax Vaccine, Adsorbed, press releases, and other documents of interest.[121]

While the internet has contributed to many improvements in our society, there are also dangers. The informational world-wide-web sites on anthrax have potential value, but they can also be the source of significant confusion and misinformation. For example, the debate over Anthrax Vaccine, Adsorbed has led to questions on the legality of Anthrax Vaccine Immunization Program, implying military personnel are duty bound to disobey it and that the mandatory program is a violation of their civil rights.[122] It is essential to sift through and gather the facts and look at both sides of a position before drawing any conclusions. In many ways, the availability of information on the internet, especially the free flow of ideas and opinions, makes critical, scientifically-based objective thought more difficult.[123]

It is important to note that the basic facts regarding the history of development of Anthrax Vaccine, Adsorbed, Michigan Biological Products Institute, BioPort, Food and Drug Administration licensure, clinical results, etc., presented on internet web sites opposed to the Anthrax Vaccine Immunization Program are usually found within links to other sites containing on-line documents. These facts and documents generally match the information presented on the Defense Department anthrax informational web site.[124] The difference is how the facts are presented, often with the insertion of subjective opinion and editorial comments, taking some point within the document referred to in the link out of context.

For example, one title says the Food and Drug Administration admits it has never received data on the long-term health effects. In reality this is a link to a letter the director of the Center for Biologics, Evaluations, and Research for the Food and Drug Administration wrote to the Executive Director for Veterans for Integrity in Government.[125] The letter responds to a series of questions, including whether or not any studies on the long-term health effects of Anthrax Vaccine, Adsorbed have been performed. The letter actually says the data has not been submitted to the Food and Drug Administration, but adds that for 28 years the vaccine had (at the time of writing) been used by veterinarians, laboratory personnel, industrial workers, and Food and Drug Administration inspectors. The clear intent of the answer is that the long-term health effects data does exist but it has not been formally submitted to the Food and Drug Administration.

One of the links on the "Anthrax Vaccine Links and Information" internet web site announces there have been British reports of outbreaks of Gulf War Syndrome after "recent" anthrax vaccinations. It references a British article entitled "Anti Bio-weapon Vaccine for troops Fails Safety Tests" from an independent British newspaper which reports newly produced lots of the British anthrax vaccine failed safety tests.[126] The article cites concerns from British Persian Gulf War veterans that the British version of the anthrax vaccine may have caused Gulf War Syndrome and that further use of the vaccine may cause more to develop symptoms. They claim many fell ill after recent vaccinations but the article provides no substantiating information. The article further alleges the lots used had expired and the shelf life had been extended several times.[127]

This link could be very misleading given the current debate about Anthrax Vaccine, Adsorbed since the article really is not about Anthrax Vaccine, Adsorbed. The British version of the anthrax vaccine is not Anthrax Vaccine, Adsorbed, is not produced either by Michigan Biological Products Institute or BioPort, does not require Food and Drug Administration licensure, and is not used in the United States. Furthermore, the Food and Drug Administration and British regulatory systems are completely separate. Yet the "Anthrax Vaccine Links and Information" site contains no statements to make this distinction.

Many who are opposed to the Anthrax Vaccine Immunization Program have attempted to connect the use of Anthrax Vaccine, Adsorbed with Gulf War Syndrome in spite of the fact that no such causal relationship has ever been demonstrated.[128] Several headings of links on the "Anthrax Vaccine Links and Information" site seem to suggest a conspiracy theory with titles like "MOU: Defense Department's & Food and Drug Administration's Secret Deal."[129] In reality the document is the memorandum of understanding outlining interagency cooperation for medical research, outlining roles, responsibilities, and reporting procedures.[130] The intent of the document is to ensure patient safety when humans are involved in medical protocol studies.

Many press release articles in the media either confuse facts, combine separate facts, or report facts in such a way as to be potentially incriminating. For example, an extensive article published in the *Phoenix New Times* states that anthrax vaccine production has been halted due to problems with the new BioPort production facilities.[131] Actually, Michigan Biological Products Institute voluntarily halted production in order to renovate the facility, then later sold the facility to BioPort. After the sale, BioPort completed renovations but has had problems obtaining Food and Drug Administration certification of the renovated facility. While both facts are true, they are not directly, nor causally, related to each other as the *Phoenix New Times* article implies. This article also attempts to raise concerns that there could be birth defects if a man who received Anthrax Vaccine, Adsorbed were to father a child.

Another example is an Associated Press article entitled, "Food and Drug Administration inspection cites problems in vaccine production."[132] A careful reading correctly indicates that the problems are with certification of the renovated facilities, required before new batches of Anthrax Vaccine, Adsorbed may be sold. But, the last sentence of the article states several anthrax vaccine lots failed Food and Drug Administration potency testing. The article does not clarify that these were older lots, none of which have been used by the Defense Department. While the last statement is true by itself, there is no attempt to prevent confusion with statements regarding the recent Food and Drug Administration facilities inspection. This could lead one not familiar with the facts to believe there is a direct relationship between the recent inspections, lots of Anthrax Vaccine, Adsorbed that failed potency testing, and the lots of vaccine currently in use by the Defense Department where, in fact, no such direct relationship exists.

Other links seem intended to provoke an emotional response, such as one with photographs of injection sites with signs of local reactions entitled "Painful Anthrax injection site photos…OUCH!" Others refer to the numerous cases of individuals at Dover Air Force Base who claim to have developed symptoms after receiving Anthrax Vaccine, Adsorbed, claiming this proves the Defense Department really knows that the vaccine is not safe. And there are links to support groups and on-line chat rooms where those opposed to the Anthrax Vaccine Immunization Program may discuss their views or tell their story.

Interestingly, there are also links to other sites opposed to the use of other types of vaccines (e.g., hepatitis B vaccine) or all vaccines in general. This suggests that those opposed to the use of Anthrax Vaccine, Adsorbed and the Anthrax Vaccine Immunization Program are part of a larger movement opposed to the use of all vaccines, promoting an anti-vaccination agenda. Other links take an alarmist approach, warning what may happen to individuals who refuse to receive Anthrax Vaccine, Adsorbed and giving advice and contact information if they "are being threatened with forcible innoculation (sic) of the Anthrax vaccine."[133]

Other examples abound and space does not permit a full analysis of all the links for and against the Defense Department's anthrax vaccine immunization effort. Suffice it to say, the wording of the headings of the links combined with selective reporting could potentially influence the opinions of readers who have not had the opportunity to familiarize themselves with all the facts. It is important for commanders and supervisors to be aware that these information sites are intentionally biased, presenting information in a way to substantiate a preconceived notion or opinion against the use of Anthrax Vaccine, Adsorbed.[134] When referring to such sites, it is worthwhile to keep the biased nature of these sites in mind and spend some extra time to read the source documents these sites claim substantiate their opinions.

At the forefront of the opposition to the Defense Department's Anthrax Vaccine Immunization Program is an emergency room physician from Maine, Dr. Meryl Nass, regarded by opponents to the program as an expert on anthrax and Anthrax Vaccine, Adsorbed.[135]   She has written a number of articles on these subjects and testified before Congress several times against the Anthrax Vaccine Immunization Program. For example, one link on the "Anthrax Vaccine Links and Information" site makes the claim that the Defense Department really does know the anthrax vaccine is not safe. It turns out the link leads to an unpublished article written by Dr. Nass about an informational meeting for 100 physicians at Fort Detrick, Maryland, in May 1999 where issues about Anthrax Vaccine, Adsorbed were discussed. Her article implies that military physicians asking policy questions about Anthrax Vaccine, Adsorbed and the Vaccine Adverse Events Reporting System proves the Defense Department does in fact know the vaccine is not safe. She ends by admonishing the readers to contact their congressional representatives.

Dr. Nass also has her own informational world-wide-web home page about anthrax.[136] The "Anthrax Vaccine Links and Information" site lists her credentials, which includes three years experience studying the anthrax outbreak in Zimbabwe.[137] She is quoted as saying as many as 10 percent of those receiving Anthrax Vaccine, Adsorbed have gotten sick, although there is no explanation of what that means—whether the symptoms were mild, moderate, severe, localized, or systemic.[138]

In 1999, Dr. Nass published an article reviewing the anthrax vaccine and its potential protective value against a biological attack with weaponized anthrax.[139] While extensively researched and documented, she cites sources that are of questionable veracity. For example, she alleges the Defense Department may have attempted to increase the potency of Anthrax Vaccine, Adsorbed by secretly adding squalene, citing herself as the source by referring to a letter she wrote to the Army Surgeon General in May 1998.[140] Based on this allegation, she implies a potential connection between Gulf War Syndrome and Defense Department vaccination programs, including Anthrax Vaccine, Adsorbed, which is the basis for most of the concern with the safety and efficacy of the vaccine.

She also states in this article "the present human anthrax vaccine probably provides only limited protection for troops facing a BW (sic) attack by anthrax."[141] She bases this assertion on the lack of controlled studies in humans that investigate the clinical effectiveness of Anthrax Vaccine, Adsorbed against inhalation anthrax during a biological attack.

Yet she presents no clinical data of her own to substantiate her claim that Anthrax Vaccine, Adsorbed may not be effective in preventing inhalation anthrax after a biological attack. In other words, in her opinion, the more than 30 years of clinical data from field trials of anthrax vaccine in workers exposed to anthrax; the absence of inhalation anthrax in the workplace since 1978; and the animal studies that demonstrate Anthrax Vaccine, Adsorbed's effectiveness in preventing inhalation anthrax, are not enough to conclude the vaccine may prevent inhalation anthrax after an attack. Instead, she implies the only way to justify using Anthrax Vaccine, Adsorbed to protect against inhalation anthrax would be to design and conduct a study in which humans are deliberately exposed to aerosolized anthrax spores.

In another document on her web site entitled "Adverse Effects: Anthrax Vaccine," Dr. Nass discusses the rates of adverse effects of Anthrax Vaccine, Adsorbed.[142] In this document, she refers to the Pittman and Tripler data discussed earlier, but generalizes the data on systemic reactions into one category. She states Pittman reported a systemic reaction rate of 43 percent and local reaction rates of 21 percent with 5 percent for moderate or severe local reactions, respectively. Referring to the Tripler report, she cites a 48 percent systemic reaction rate and local reaction rates of 80 percent overall, but does not report the rate for moderate and severe local reactions. She cites as her sources the General Accounting Office Congressional testimony given 29 April 1999 and 12 October 1999.

During his 29 April 1999 testimony before Congress, Kwai-Cheung Chan, Director, Special Studies and Evaluations, National Security and International Affairs Division, the General Accounting Office, referred to data from four safety studies involving Anthrax Vaccine, Adsorbed.[143] Included are tables clearly distinguishing between mild versus moderate/severe systemic reactions. Whereas Dr. Nass claims the Pittman study showed an occurrence rate of 43 percent for systemic reactions to Anthrax Vaccine, Adsorbed, the Pittman study actually distinguishes between occurrence rates for mild (29 percent) and moderate/severe (14 percent) systemic reactions. Similarly, the Tripler study, in which Dr. Nass says there was an occurrence rate of 48 percent for systemic reactions, actually reported that the rate of moderate or severe systemic reactions was 5 percent while the rate for mild systemic reactions was 43 percent.[144]

The numbers involved in the Pittman and Tripler studies are very low, roughly 500 for each. Recall that the Canadian Armed Forces study involved 547 participants, but in that study the occurrence rates for systemic reactions were lower than the rates listed in the Food and Drug Administration package insert for Anthrax Vaccine, Adsorbed. Otherd studies already cited, involving tens of thousands of participants, also document systemic reaction rates that are much lower, especially for moderate and severe reactions, suggesting the Pittman and Tripler studies may not be statistically valid. Distinguishing between mild versus moderate and severe systemic reactions and accounting for the low numbers involved in these two studies is important. Not making these distinctions, plus attempting to build a case on data that may be statistically limited, could inadvertently mislead those not familiar with the actual studies to conclude the risk from Anthrax Vaccine, Adsorbed is higher than is actually the case.

Dr. Nass, in her article on adverse effects, is highly critical of the effectiveness and accuracy of the Vaccine Adverse Events Reporting System data for Anthrax Vaccine, Adsorbed and the Anthrax Vaccine Immunization Program, believing that the rate of reporting data by Defense Department health care workers is low. She alleges that Defense Department health care workers and physicians were ordered not to report any but the most severe reactions and not to report any symptoms or reactions not specifically listed in the Food and Drug Administration package insert for Anthrax Vaccine, Adsorbed.[145] She gives no source or substantiating documentation for this allegation. She also states that the package insert for Anthrax Vaccine, Adsorbed, as required by the Food and Drug Administration, was written using only information from the Brachman study vaccine, the precursor of Anthrax Vaccine, Adsorbed. And she asserts the Brachman study is the only study with "published" reaction rates for anthrax vaccine.

The purpose of the Vaccine Adverse Events Reporting System is to gather ongoing, long-term data on potential adverse reactions due to vaccines that were not identified during limited clinical trials. For example, if the incidence of a particular reaction or severe systemic effect occurring is one in a million, then several hundred thousand or even several million doses may have to be administered before that reaction would be observed. In reality, such extensive, long-term studies are not possible during clinical trials. Furthermore, if evidence exists that the vaccine will prevent more disease and save more lives than any harm caused by the vaccine, it may be regarded as unethical to withhold the vaccine from market to conduct long-term studies. The Food and Drug Administration instituted the Vaccine Adverse Events Reporting System to continue to collect data over the long-term, after vaccines are released for sale, to look for extremely rare adverse effects even though initial studies indicate a vaccine is safe and effective.

The Vaccine Adverse Events Reporting System is a passive reporting system, meaning that individuals must take the initiative to file a report.[146] There is no one that actively calls or surveys vaccinated individuals to see if they developed any symptoms. In some cases this could be a disadvantage, leading to low reporting rates. Also, it is not possible just by using this data to establish that a particular vaccine actually caused an event. But, through the identification of possible trends over the long term, Vaccine Adverse Events Reporting System data is useful to direct new clinical studies to establish causality.

Several facets have been built into the Vaccine Adverse Events Reporting System to facilitate reporting. For example, anyone, including patients and families, may report any symptom suspected due to a vaccine. In addition, medical personnel are routinely reminded through extensive educational programs about the need to report to this database. Furthermore, medical personnel are required to report adverse effects due to vaccines to the manufacturer who is then required to report those events to Vaccine Adverse Events Reporting System.[147]

The Vaccine Adverse Events Reporting System receives over 12,000 reports of possible adverse reactions to vaccines each year. Fifteen percent are considered serious, including those that are life-threatening, result in hospitalization, missed work, or permanent disability. It should be noted that for some childhood vaccines, more reports of potential adverse effects from the vaccine are filed each year than the number of reported cases of the disease the vaccine is designed to prevent.[148] This cumulative evidence suggests that, contrary to the criticisms of Anthrax

Vaccine Immunization Program opponents, the Vaccine Adverse Events Reporting System is highly successful.

The Defense Department has reiterated to medical personnel that they should report any events they feel may be due to Anthrax Vaccine, Adsorbed. There is no documentation that the Defense Department instructed medical personnel to file a report only when they observe the side effects and reactions listed in the Food and Drug Administration package insert.[149] Instead, the Defense Department encourages all medical personnel to report all events potentially thought to be related to Anthrax Vaccine, Adsorbed and requires them to report to the Vaccine Adverse Events Reporting System all adverse reactions potentially associated with the vaccine resulting in hospitalization or loss of more than 24 hours duty.[150] Additionally, in 1999, the Air Force Surgeon General directed that any adverse events even suspected by medical personnel to be related to Anthrax Vaccine, Adsorbed will be reported to the Vaccine Adverse Events Reporting System.[151] Dr. Nass' allegations that Defense Department physicians are prohibited from filing reports to the Vaccine Adverse Events Reporting System on any potential Anthrax Vaccine, Adsorbed related event are completely unfounded, ignoring the fact that such prohibitions may be illegal.

As already discussed, licensure of Anthrax Vaccine, Adsorbed (and the information for the package insert) was based on both the Brachman study and data collected by the Centers for Disease Control and Prevention over a 10-year period on the use of Anthrax Vaccine, Adsorbed in workers considered at risk for exposure to anthrax spores. Furthermore, the Brachman study is not the only place where data on the safety and efficacy of Anthrax Vaccine, Adsorbed has been published. As already noted in this paper, there have been numerous other studies (e.g., the Centers for Disease Control and Prevention study) on the safety and efficacy of Anthrax Vaccine, Adsorbed conducted over several years involving tens of thousands of human subjects.[152]

Although not all of these studies are individually published as peer-reviewed articles (like the Brachman study), the data collected by these studies has been examined by review panels and published in several articles that have undergone the peer-review process.[153] Stating that the Brachman study contains the "ONLY published adverse reaction rates" without acknowledging these other sources of data in the peer-reviewed literature is misleading.[154]

Another concern raised by opponents to the Anthrax Vaccine Immunization Program is that adversaries might develop strains of anthrax that are resistant to Anthrax Vaccine, Adsorbed.[155] Some base this on the fact that strains of anthrax have been developed that are resistant to antibiotics. Also, there have been reports that anthrax strains have been developed that may render the Russian-developed live attenuated vaccine ineffective.[156] Neither of these reports mean that a strain of anthrax has been produced that is resistant to Anthrax Vaccine, Adsorbed.

First, it must be pointed out that developing resistance to antibiotics is not the same as developing resistance to vaccines. Antibiotics (biochemicals produced in nature or synthesized in laboratories that are toxic to bacteria) are completely different from antibodies (complex proteins produced by the inoculated individual's immune cells) that result from vaccination. Bacteria commonly develop resistance to antibiotics through several naturally occurring mechanisms, resulting in the antibiotic (such as penicillin or tetracycline) no longer being toxic to the bacteria.

Anthrax Vaccine, Adsorbed, however, induces the inoculated individual to produce antibodies against protective antigen, which also is a protein. In order for anthrax to develop a resistance to the vaccine, the bacteria's genetic code for protective antigen would have to be altered in such a way so the bacteria produces an altered version of protective antigen that the antibodies cannot recognize. But the protective antigen would still have to retain its functional ability to combine with the host's cells and the other anthrax toxins (which are also proteins made by anthrax bacteria) to produce disease.

An adversary intent on producing a strain of anthrax resistant to Anthrax Vaccine, Adsorbed would, therefore, need to possess highly sophisticated and very expensive genetic engineering capabilities. Needless to say, any genetics program intended to alter anthrax to change the characteristics of protective antigen would be a costly monumental undertaking and well beyond the reach of most potential adversaries. Not surprisingly, there is no documentation that a strain of anthrax consistently resistant to Anthrax Vaccine, Adsorbed in all species has been produced.[157]

No vaccine is perfect, meaning that no vaccine is 100 percent safe and effective. But, as has been presented, the clinical evidence suggests Anthrax Vaccine, Adsorbed is safe and effective—probably safer with lower rates of side effects than other vaccines in use today. But, even though Anthrax Vaccine, Adsorbed is safe and effective, that does not mean there is no room for improvement regarding vaccinations against anthrax.[158]

The requirement for six inoculations with Anthrax Vaccine, Adsorbed creates a significant logistical problem for the Defense Department's Anthrax Vaccine Immunization Program, especially as supplies of currently re-tested and approved lots of vaccine are running low. But, the current requirement for six inoculations is in accordance with the Food and Drug Administration licensure of Anthrax Vaccine, Adsorbed and probably won't change unless studies are done to confirm that the vaccine provides protection with fewer doses. Newer vaccines that require fewer doses to confer immunity have been developed but have not been approved for use by the Food and Drug Administration.[159] The 30 percent rate of occurrence of local reactions ideally could be lower, although it has already been pointed out that this rate is already lower than other vaccines currently required by the Defense Department.

A major challenge is how to demonstrate an individual has developed adequate immunity against anthrax after vaccination either with Anthrax Vaccine, Adsorbed or a newer anthrax vaccine without exposing the individual to aerosolized anthrax spores. As discussed previously, it is not ethical to expose individuals to aerosolized anthrax spores to see if the vaccine prevents development of inhalation anthrax. Using animal models may or may not be useful since species differ in their sensitivity to anthrax and differences in their immune systems may alter the efficacy with which anthrax vaccines confer immunity. Measuring the level of antibodies an individual has circulating in the blood against protective antigen has been shown to be a very unreliable measurement of immunity against anthrax. The next best approach would be to develop a test that could be administered to the individual to indicate the degree of immunity. Currently no such test exists, which is one reason why the Food and Drug Administration recommends a series of six shots of Anthrax Vaccine, Adsorbed with an annual booster. With such a test, individuals could be screened and only those with inadequate immune responses would require supplemental inoculations, potentially decreasing the required number of doses of vaccine.

It should be reiterated, however, that even though there is room for improvement, none of these issues negate the current value and effectiveness of Anthrax Vaccine, Adsorbed. In contrast, Dr. Nass warns that submitting to the Anthrax Vaccine Immunization Program is like playing Russian Roulette with your life since there is the possibility there could be side effects.[160] But, following this line of reasoning, one should never receive any vaccine (or take any other medication or undergo any medical procedure for that matter) since all vaccines have risks associated with their use and no vaccine is totally risk-free.

Dr. Nass believes there should be more emphasis on using alternatives to vaccination with Anthrax Vaccine, Adsorbed to protect troops from anthrax. For example, she suggests there should be more emphasis on the use of protective equipment. The problem with this approach is, due to the lack of real-time detection capability, there is no way for personnel to know when they need to wear the protective equipment, meaning they would have to wear it continually to be effective.

Dr. Nass also expresses concern that immunizing troops against anthrax may provoke an adversary to simply pick another agent.[161] As previously discussed, other biological agents are more difficult to weaponize and the likelihood that other agents would be used in an attack instead of anthrax is much lower.

Dr. Nass also expresses hope that creation of and adherence to better international biological weapons conventions, including provisions for surprise inspections and stiff penalties for non-compliance, will improve nonproliferation efforts. Sadly, there is ample historical evidence that several signatory nations have already violated current nonproliferation arms control agreements like the Nuclear Nonproliferation Treaty, in spite of provisions for "on-site" inspections.[162]

Another writer goes as far as to suggest there should not be any vaccinations of Defense Department personnel until an anthrax-based biological weapon is actually used, even though he acknowledges that historical precedent exists to justify concern that anthrax could be used as a political tool.[163] This reactionary approach ignores the ready availability of anthrax spores and that anthrax is easily weaponized and that some states of concern like Iraq, have been proved to have done so.

Recall also, that there are limitations associated with constant use of personal protective gear, that there are limitations with gathering intelligence to provide advanced warning of an attack, and that no means exists to detect reliably that an attack with anthrax is occurring.

Considering that international conventions historically have failed to prevent proliferation of biological weapons (even in spite of on-site inspections), and that it takes time for an individual to develop an immunity against anthrax after vaccination, it becomes apparent that waiting until an attack is imminent before immunizing personnel would not only be ineffective, but dangerous.[164] Consequently, immunization against anthrax before an attack becomes imminent is still our best pro-active defense to protect personnel from attacks using anthrax-based biological weapons.

At Dover Air Force Base, Delaware, the number of individuals reporting adverse reactions after inoculation with Anthrax Vaccine, Adsorbed appears to exceed the rate one would expect based on the published literature. A list of many of the symptoms reported can be found on the world-wide-web.[165] There are several problems, however, trying to make a connection between these symptoms and Anthrax Vaccine, Adsorbed. First of all, there is no discernible pattern to the symptoms. The time of onset between vaccination and the onset of symptoms is highly variable, ranging from a few hours to months. The listings on the web site do not indicate if these patients got better, except in one or two cases.

From a statistical perspective, after almost 40 years of clinical experience with Anthrax Vaccine, Adsorbed, plus several studies documenting its safety, why would there be this sudden cluster of cases at Dover? By way of contrast, the U.S. Army Medical Research Institute of Infectious Diseases tracked 1,590 individuals who received 10,451 doses of Anthrax Vaccine, Adsorbed over several years, documenting rates of adverse events no higher than those listed in the Food and Drug Administration package insert and no loss of duty.[166]

With no recurrent pattern of symptoms, and no consistent temporal relation of the development of symptoms to inoculation with Anthrax

Vaccine, Adsorbed, it is extremely difficult to claim the cases at Dover prove Anthrax Vaccine, Adsorbed is the cause.[167] In addition, the rate of occurrence of any disease (for example thyroid disease) in vaccinated personnel at Dover is equal to or less than the rate of occurrence of the same disease in unvaccinated individuals. And the rate of occurrence of individual symptoms in personnel vaccinated with Anthrax Vaccine, Adsorbed is no higher than the rate expected when vaccinating personnel with any other vaccine, further complicating claims that Anthrax Vaccine, Adsorbed caused the symptoms.[168]

Without a doubt it would be wrong to trivialize the symptoms these patients are experiencing. The symptoms are very real and must be addressed in a compassionate, professional manner. But, the fact that these individuals are having symptoms and the fact that they received Anthrax Vaccine, Adsorbed does not prove that the vaccine caused the symptoms. In contrast, it is more likely these individuals would have developed the symptoms from which they currently suffer even if they had not received the vaccine.

The debate over Anthrax Vaccine, Adsorbed has led to introduction of a bill in Congress that would suspend the Defense Department's Anthrax Vaccine Immunization Program.[169] Much of the language of the bill cites language similar to the language found on the "Anthrax Vaccine Links and Information" site. The bill would also prohibit the gathering of any data whatsoever on adverse effects potentially related to Anthrax Vaccine, Adsorbed.

This prohibition is indeed unfortunate for three reasons. First, there is nothing unethical about collecting data while the Anthrax Vaccine Immunization Program is in effect. Second, the Defense Department would not be able to collect the vast amount of valuable data that could be used to resolve the issues and concerns that led to the introduction of the bill. Third, the bill ignores the relative risks of not vaccinating Defense Department personnel (including the real risk that military personnel could be attacked with an anthrax weapon and the lethality of inhalation anthrax) versus the large amount of clinical data documenting Anthrax Vaccine, Adsorbed's safety and efficacy.

Lieutenant General (retired) James T. Scott recently wrote an editorial which, arguably, does more to place the entire controversy over the

Defense Department's anthrax vaccination into proper perspective than any other work examined in this paper.[170] He states that both sides share the blame for escalating this debate out of proportion. The Defense Department could have done better stating its case in the beginning for a comprehensive vaccination program in peacetime. The Defense Department's credibility had already been damaged by how it handled the Agent Orange and Gulf War Syndrome issues. This problem is exacerbated by the chronic under-funding of the military health care system that is eroding away what little confidence beneficiaries may have in military health care. And the Defense Department failed to anticipate the effect the internet would have on spreading dis-information campaigns against the Anthrax Vaccine Immunization Program.

To the opponents who are also Service members, Scott writes that it is time to find out the facts. He states Service members concerned over the Defense Department's Anthrax Vaccine Immunization Program should be sure the information they possess is based on solid facts. He admonishes those opposed to the Immunization Program to ask themselves if they are only concerned with the safety and efficacy of Anthrax Vaccine, Adsorbed or if their concerns run much deeper—that their opposition to the Anthrax Vaccine Immunization Program may reflect that they have lost complete confidence in the military system. If so, it may be time for them to find a career outside the military.

To military leaders and supervisors, Scott says the controversy over the Defense Department's Anthrax Vaccine Immunization Program is not a test of leadership. The ability to talk subordinates into vaccination versus court-martialing those who refuse is a false test and misses the point. The real issue is how they will restore their subordinates' confidence in the mission, the chain of command, the unit, and each other. This confidence should be based on "rational explanations based on credible evidence."[171] In an all-volunteer force of such high quality people, the "men and women who serve in our armed forces deserve no less."[172]

IX. Conclusions and Recommendations

The current anthrax vaccine, Anthrax Vaccine, Adsorbed, is a licensed vaccine and has been demonstrated to be clinically safe and effective for preventing inhalation anthrax after exposure to anthrax spores. Based on the findings of the 1985 advisory review panel examining the safety and efficacy of Anthrax Vaccine, Adsorbed, the Food and Drug Administration categorized the vaccine as a "Category 1 (safe, effective, and not misbranded) vaccine."[173] In spite of the existing documentation of the safety and efficacy of Anthrax Vaccine, Adsorbed, the Defense Department continues to ask outside consultants and panels to review the evidence documenting the safety and efficacy of the vaccine. For example, recently the Defense Department asked the Institute of Medicine to review all available data on Anthrax Vaccine, Adsorbed.[174] One would be hard pressed to identify another vaccine in use today that has undergone more scrutiny than Anthrax Vaccine, Adsorbed.

There are significant issues with Anthrax Vaccine, Adsorbed that should be addressed, including the current dosage regimen (requiring six doses with annual booster shots), the inability to specifically measure the level of immunity an individual may already possess, and the occurrence of local reactions in 30 percent of those who are vaccinated. In spite of these issues, there is no clinical evidence that the Defense Department's Anthrax Vaccine Immunization Program to vaccinate personnel considered to be at risk for exposure to anthrax should be stopped. The risk of serious adverse reactions or permanent injury from Anthrax Vaccine, Adsorbed is no higher than (and, in fact, is probably lower than) that for any other vaccine commonly in use in the general population today. In contrast, the risks to military personnel from the threat of attack with an anthrax-based biological weapon, plus the high lethality of inhalation anthrax, far outweigh the risks associated with vaccination.

The large number of doses of Anthrax Vaccine, Adsorbed required to establish immunity, plus the annual requirement for a booster, create significant problems in terms of logistics and costs for the Defense Department to complete the Anthrax Vaccine Immunization Program and vaccinate all Defense Department personnel, especially in light of dwindling supplies of vaccine. Ideally, a reliable test to measure an individual's immunity against anthrax should be developed. To ease the burden, only personnel expected to deploy to areas where the risk for potential use of weaponized anthrax is highest should be vaccinated. Military personnel not expected to deploy to these areas are at no greater risk for exposure to weaponized anthrax spores than the general population of the United States, and need not be vaccinated. This is consistent with consensus panel recommendations that there is no requirement to vaccinate the entire population of the U.S. since the risk of exposure to weaponized anthrax for any given community within the U.S. is extremely low.[175]

The U.S. Army Medical Research Institute of Infections Diseases completed pre-clinical research on a next-generation anthrax vaccine several years ago. The new recombinant vaccine is now in advanced clinical development. Unfortunately, Food and Drug Administration approval of a new vaccine is still several years away. In the meantime, long-term data collection studies should continue in order to document further the safety of Anthrax Vaccine, Adsorbed and attempt to identify extremely rare adverse effects which may only become apparent after millions of doses of vaccine have been administered. The Defense Department should also continue with programs to provide long-term follow-up to individuals claiming to have developed symptoms after receiving Anthrax Vaccine, Adsorbed. These patients' symptoms are real and they deserve compassionate, professional medical care.

Continuance of the Anthrax Vaccine Immunization Program should include an aggressive, active educational and informational program designed to address concerns at all levels, from the top leadership down to the installation level. The Defense Department web site and its links to other Service-specific web sites are excellent but passive, meaning they depend on people going to these sites to get the facts. What is needed is an active education program where information is actively taken out to the troops.

Defense Department programs actively promoting education of all military personnel, using the information on the Defense Department internet web site, could significantly alleviate the suspicions and doubts currently surrounding the Anthrax Vaccine Immunization Program. Commander and supervisor involvement at every level of command is essential to begin rebuilding the confidence military personnel should have in their chains of command.

Commanders and supervisors should be aware of the biased nature of informational internet web sites opposed to the Anthrax Vaccine Immunization Program, emphasizing to their personnel the importance of basing any conclusions about Anthrax Vaccine, Adsorbed or the Anthrax Vaccine Immunization Program on all the facts. Such proactive educational efforts should prove useful to reverse any negative trends and perceptions emanating from the Defense Department's handling of the Agent Orange and Gulf War Syndrome issues. The Anthrax Vaccine Immunization Program should be viewed as an opportunity for the Department of Defense to demonstrate its commitment to maintaining the health and safety of Service personnel while countering any threat to our nation's security from anthrax-based mass-casualty weapons.

Notes

1. Major Sonny Bates' home page is found at http://www.majorbates.com/

2. The Air Force eventually allowed Major Bates to resign his commission. See Representative Dan Burton, Letter to Secretary of Defense William Cohen, 12 May, 2000, on-line, internet, 27 August 2000, available from http://www.house.gov/reform/letters/cohen.5.12.00.pdf.

3. Dr. Robert C. Myers, Statement Presented to the Subcommittee on National Security, Veterans Affairs, and International Relations, 29 April 1999, on-line, internet, 11 February 2000, available from http://www.bioportcorp.com/testimony_of_drmyers.htm.

4. This is the approach used in an article recently published by Mazzuchi, et al. In this article the authors emphasize that the decision to immunize is a command policy decision even though maintaining the health of the Service members is the primary objective. See John F. Mazzuichi, Robert G. Claypool, Kenneth C. Hyams, David Trump, James Riddle, Relford E. Patterson, Sue Bailey, "Protecting the Health of U.S. Military Forces: A National Obligation," *Aviation, Space, and Environmental Medicine,* 71, no. 3 March 2000, 260-265.

5. "Peer-reviewed" refers to the process major medical journals use to decide if submissions are worthy of publication. Normally, the lead investigator submits a manuscript for consideration to the editorial board. The editorial board then selects members of the board (unknown to the author of the manuscript) to review the article to see if it meets stringent criteria such as scientific process, experimental design, analysis of the data, discussion, and conclusions. Some journal editorial boards "blind" the editorial reviewers and authors from each other so the reviewers and authors do not know whose work is being reviewed to make the review process more objective. The peer-review process is considered to be the most effective means of assuring quality publications in the medical literature. It should be noted that medical textbooks are not peer-reviewed although there is an editor to whom writers of the individual book chapters submit their manuscripts. Therefore, publishing in a textbook is not considered to be as significant as publication in a peer-reviewed journal.

6. Numerous extensive reviews of the disease process of anthrax, the vaccine, and the threat weaponized anthrax poses to United States military personnel already exist in the literature. Many are cited in this paper.

7. Numerous countries, including those who are signatories of the Biological Weapons and Toxins Convention (including the former Soviet Union and Iraq) are known to have offensive biological weapons development programs, including development of weapons using anthrax as the agent. Major D. L. Clements, in an interesting study, concludes that overt use of tactical biological agents on the battlefield is

unlikely due to difficulty in hiding the identity of the attacker and the risk of overwhelming response. Biological attacks against United States forces overseas are, in his opinion, more likely to be on a small scale by terrorist groups. He identifies anthrax as the ideal biological warfare agent and concludes its use by terrorists or covert operators (such as special forces) against U.S. forces either in the U.S. or overseas is highly plausible, especially during deployments. See Major David Lee Clement, "A Determination of the Military Significance of Modern Biological Warfare," Master's Thesis, U.S. Army Command and General Staff College, Ft. Leavenworth, KS, 1993, 70, 79. See also Thomas V. Inglesby, et al, "Anthrax as a Biological Weapon," *Journal of the American Medical Association*, 281, no. 18, 12 May 1999, 1735-1745. This article states that anthrax is one of the most serious agents that could be used as a biological weapon, presenting a clinical discussion of anthrax to demonstrate why it would make such an effective weapon. Mazzuchi, et al, op. cit., 261. For more information related to the threat anthrax poses as a potential biological weapon, the reader is referred to the United States Air Force Counterproliferation Center's world-wide-web site at http://www.au.af.mil/au/awc/awcgate/awc-cps.htm which is updated regularly and contains numerous links to other important sites on this topic.

8. For more detailed information, the reader is referred to the Defense Department's informational world-wide-web site addressing anthrax vaccination at http://www.anthrax.osd.mil/. This site includes several links to papers, covering a variety of issues related to the anthrax vaccine. There are also several web sites outlining the reasons against the Defense Department's anthrax vaccination program. The most prominent and complete with numerous links to other sites is http://www.dallasnw.quik.com/cyberella/index.htm. It is important to note that these sites present nearly identical historical, clinical, and factual information. Where these sites differ is how they interpret the information and what conclusions they draw.

9. The Gram stain is a special stain invented by and named for Christian Gram. Bob A. Freeman, "The Physical and Chemical Structure of Bacteria," *Burrows Textbook of Microbiology*, 21st Edition, (Philadelphia, PA: W.B. Saunders Company, 1979), 25. Used to classify bacteria when looking through a microscope. Gram positive bacteria absorb a crystal violet stain, turning it deep violet in color, whereas Gram negative bacteria do not.

10. Terry C. Dixon et al, "Anthrax," *The New England Journal of Medicine,* 341, no. 11, 9 September 1999: 815-826.

11 R. K. Holmes, "Diptheria, Other Cornybacterial Infections, and Anthrax," in *Harrison's Principles of Internal Medicine,* 14th edition, eds. Anthony S Fauci, M.D. et al. (New York, NY: McGraw-Hill, 1998), 897. See also, Phillip S. Brachman, "Anthrax," in *Infectious Diseases* 3rd edition, edited by Paul D. Hoeprich, M.D. (Philadelphia, PA: Harper&Row, Publishers, 1983), 939.

12 Thomas V. Inglesby et al, "Anthrax as a Biological Weapon," *Journal of the American Medical Association,* 281, no. 18, 12 May, 1999, 1735-1745.

13. "Anthrax History: What You Need to Know," on-line, internet, 11 February 2000, available from http://www.anthrax.osd.mil/.

14. Daniel Lew, "Bacilluus Anthracis," in *Principles and Practice of Infectious Diseases*, 4th ed., vol. 2, eds. Gerald l. Mandell, John E. Bennett, and Raphael Dolin, editors, (New York, NY: Churchill Livingstone, 1995), 1885.

15. Kenneth W. Hedlund, "Anthrax Toxin: History and Recent Advances and Perspectives," *Journal of Toxicology* 11, no. 1, 1992, 41-88.

16. Holmes, op. cit., 897.

17. Brachman, op. cit., 944.

18. Inglesby, 1736.

19. Holmes, op. cit., 897.

20. Brachman, op. cit., 940.

21. Ibid., 943.

22. Ibid., 942.

23. Inglesby, op. cit., 1737.

24. Dixon, op. cit., 819.

25. Inglesby, 1737.

26. Ibid., 1774.

27. Ibid., 1736-1737.

28. Ibid., 1743-1744. See also a paper written as part of a series entitled "The Military Readiness Project," sponsored by the Family Research Council. See George T. Havrilak, "The Pentagon's Anthrax Vaccination Immunization Program," (no date), n.p., on-line, internet, 9 September 2000, available from http://www.frc.org/military/mp99k1mf.html.

29. Dixon, op. cit., 818.

30. "Hemorrhagic meningitis" refers to inflammation of the protective coverings of the brain and spinal cord with associated bleeding.

31. Ibid., 819.

32. Arthur M. Friedlander, "Anthrax," in Textbook of Military Medicine: Medical Aspects of Chemical and Biological Warfare, eds. Brigadier General Russ Zajtchuk and Ronald F. Belamy, (Washington, DC: TMM Publications, 1997), 470.

33. Ibid., 815-818. See also, Hedlund, op. cit., 53.

34. Antibiotics and antibodies are completely different. Antibiotics are chemicals not produced by the body that either kill or inhibit the growth of bacteria. Antibodies are complex proteins produced by the body that circulate in the blood and recognize foreign substances. Bacterial resistance to antibiotics means that bacterial growth is not affected by that particular antibiotic. It does not imply the bacteria are resistant to antibodies.

35. Inglesby, op. cit., 1741.

36. "Approved of CIPRO® For Use After Exposure to Inhalational Anthrax,"" 31 August 2000, on-line, internet, 3 November 2000, available from http://www.fda.gov/bbs/topics/ANSWERS/ANS01030.html.

37. Ideally, the antibiotics should be administered intravenously and later switched to oral medications if the patient remains asymptomatic. But, if there are large numbers of patients or limited medical facilities, oral administration is acceptable. Antibiotic treatment should be continued either for 60 days or until the possibility of exposure to anthrax has been completely and positively excluded through testing. If the anthrax vaccine is available and possible exposure to anthrax confirmed, it is reasonable to give these patients the anthrax vaccine. If these patients remain asymptomatic, then the course of antibiotics may be reduced to 30 to 45 days. Inglesby, op. cit., 1741-1743.

38. There are two different types of anthrax vaccine in existence today for human use. ("An Assessment of the Safety of the Anthrax Vaccine: A Letter Report," 30 March, 2000; on-line, internet, 12 August 2000, available from http://www.nap.edu/html/anthrax_vaccine/.) Vaccines manufactured by filtering and purifying protective antigen (such as AVA) are used in the West, primarily by the U.S. and the United Kingdom. The former Soviet Union manufactured an anthrax vaccine using live attenuated (weakened) anthrax spores. This type of vaccine is not available in the West. Although the efficacy of the live, attenuated spore vaccine has been reported to be higher than protective antigen based vaccines, see Hedlund, op. cit., 64. See also, Meryl Nass, "Anthrax Vaccine," *New Vaccines and New Vaccine Technology,* 13, No. 1, March 1999, 187-208. Nass writes that an obvious concern related to using this type of vaccine is that the live spores, although weakened, could still cause anthrax. See Inglesby, op. cit., 1740.

39. In addition to AVA, there have been a number of experimental anti-anthrax vaccines developed but not necessarily tested or released for use in humans. All anti-anthrax vaccines developed in some way center on provoking an immunogenic response to PA. See Hedlund, op. cit., 64-68.

40. Ibid., 67, 76.

41. Arthur M. Friedlander, Phillip R. Pittman, and Gerald W. Parker, "Anthrax Vaccine: Evidence for Safety and Efficacy Against Inhalation Anthrax," *Journal of the American Medical Association* 282, no. 22, 8 Dec, 1999, 2104-2106.

42. In large doses and with repeated exposure formaldehyde may cause cancer. But there is no evidence that repeated doses of trace amounts of formaldehyde when used as a preservative in vaccines is harmful.

43. "Anthrax Vaccine – Ingredients," n.p.; on-line, internet, 11 February 2000, available from http://www.anthrax.osd.mil/.

44. "Accusations – Squalene," n.p.; on-line internet, 11 February 2000, available from http://www.anthrax.osd.mil/oldavip/qna/SQUALENE.HTM.

45. Squalene actually occurs naturally in humans and is a precursor in the synthesis of cholesterol. Squalene is also found in large amounts in deep-sea shark liver. There are currently several health food supplemental products on the market containing squalene. Proponents claim squalene improves the delivery of oxygen to cells and facilitates the clearance of metabolic toxins. For more information see http://www.takari.com/prima.html and http://www.squalene.net/history.htm. A study reported by Asa et al. claims to have found that squalene antibodies are only found in the blood of people suffering from Gulf War Syndrome. This claim forms the basis of several press reports in the mainstream media accusing that the Department of Defense secretly added squalene to AVA. (Pamala B. Asa, Yon Cao, Robert F. Garry, "Antibodies to Squalene in Gulf War Syndrome," *Experimental and Molecular Pathology* 68, no. 1 (February 2000), 55-64.) It is very important to note that this study is poorly constructed and has been refuted due to insufficient numbers of subjects in the study population and lack of sufficient control groups. In addition, the authors themselves caution in the article that the results of their study do not establish that squalene was used in AVA or any other vaccine during the Persian Gulf War.

46. Meryl Nass, "Anthrax Vaccine Safety and Efficacy: Response to the Army Surgeon General Ronald Blanck's Posting," (4 May ,1998), n.p.; on-line, internet, 15 February 2000, available from http://www.dallasnw.quik.com/cyberella/Anthrax/safety4.html.

47. Karen Jowers, Unusual Compound Detected in Samples of Anthrax Vaccine," *Air Force Times*, 61, Issue 11, 9 October 2000, 28

48. "Information About the Anthrax Vaccine and the Anthrax Vaccine Immunization Program (AVIP)," 15 October 2000; on-line, internet, 2 November 2000, available from http://www.anthrax.osd.mil/HTML interface/default.html.

49. A study reported by Asa, et. al., claims to have found that squalene antibodies are only found in the blood of people suffering from Gulf War Syndrome. This claim forms the basis of several press reports in the mainstream media accusing that the Department of Defense secretly added squalene to Anthrax Vaccine, Adsorbed. See Pamala B. Asa, Yon Cao, Robert F. Garry, "Antibodies to Squalene in Gulf War Syndrome*," Experimental and Molecular Pathology*, 68, no. 1, February 2000, 55-64. It is very important to note that this study is poorly constructed and has been refuted due to insufficient numbers of subject in the study population and lack of sufficient control

groups. In addition, the authors themselves caution in the article that the results of their study do not establish that squalene was used in Anthrax Vaccine, Adsorbed or any other vaccine during the Persian Gulf War.

50. Meryl Nass, "Anthrax Vaccine Safety and Efficacy: Response to the Army Surgeon General Ronald Blanck's Posting," 4 May 1998; on-line, internet, 15 February 2000, available from http://www.dallasnw.quik.com/syberella/Anthrax/safety4.html.

51. The first anthrax vaccine was produced in the 1800s by Louis Pasteur for use in animals. It was the first vaccine ever developed to protect against bacterial infection, making anthrax the first disease for which a vaccine was ever produced. Anthrax is probably the most studied and scrutinized of any bacterial infectious disease process. "Anthrax Vaccine Immunization Program," on-line, internet, 11 February 2000, available from http://www.anthrax.osd.mil/.

52. PS Brachman, et al., "Field Evaluation of a Human Anthrax Vaccine," *American Journal of Public Health,* 62, 1962, 632-645.

53. *Federal Register,* 50, No. 240, 13 December, 1985, Part II, 51002-51117; on-line, internet. Available from http://www.anthrax.osd.mil/oldavip/FedReg1.htm. See also, Friedlander, "Anthrax Vaccine: Evidence for Safety and Efficacy Against Inhalation Anthrax," 2104. See also, Meryl Nass, "Anthrax Vaccine," New Vaccines and New Vaccine Technology, 13 no. 1, March 1999, 187-208.

54. "Anthrax Vaccine – Overview," on-line, internet, 11 Feb 2000, available from http://www.anthrax.osd.mil/oldavip/qna/OVERVIEW.HTM.

55. Friedlander, op. cit., 2104.

56. Myers, op. cit.

57. Ibid.

58. "Anthrax Vaccine, Adsorbed Stockpile Analysis – Supplemental Testing Needed and/or Resolvable FDA Issues, " 13 November 1998, n.p.: on-line Internet, 15 February 2000, available from http://www.anthraxvaccine.org/suppdocs/doc14.htm.

59. Myers, op. cit.

60. Department of Defense Press Release: 14 December, 1999; on-line internet, 11 February 2000, available from http://www.bioport.com/release12-14-99.htm.

61. Fuad El-Hibri, CEO of BioPort Corporation, Statement Presented to the Subcommittee on National Security, Veterans Affairs, and International Relations, 30 June 1999; on-line, internet, 11 February 2000, available from http://www.bioportcorp.com/El-HibriOral_Test_6-30.htm.

62. Department of Defense Press Release: 14 December, 1999.

63. Rudi Williams, "Short Supply Forces Anthrax Vaccination Slowdown," *American Forces Press Service,* 12 July 2000; on-line, internet, 26 August 2000, available from http://www.defenselink.mil/news/Jul2000/n07122000_20007124.html.

64. Myer, op. cit.

65. Department of Defense Release, 14 December 1999.

66. Ibid.

67. "Accusations – Squalene," op. cit.

68. "Department of Defense Information About the Anthrax Vaccine and the Anthrax Vaccine Immunization Program (AVIP)," 23 June 2000; on-line, internet, 26 August 2000, available from http://www.anthrax.osd.mil/Site_Files/Ed_products/Infopaper/Infopaper.htm.

69. William S. Cohen, "Anthrax Vaccination Slowdown," 10 July, 2000; on-line, internet, 26 August 2000, available from http://www.anthrax.osd.mil/Site_Files/AVIPslowdown/video_text.htm.

70. Todd Silver, "Federal Vaccine Manufacture Weighed: Pending Shortage of Anthrax Preparation Finds Congress Dissatisfied with the Status Quo," *U.S. Medicine,* 36, No. 8, August 2000, 47, 49-50.

71. Brachman, "Field Evaluation of a Human Anthrax Vaccine," op. cit.

72. Nass, "Anthrax Vaccine," op. cit., 189.

73. Myers, op. cit.

74. Ibid.

75. *Federal Register*, op. cit.

76. Susan S. Ellenberg, Director, Division of Biostatistics and Epidemiology, Center for Biologics Evaluation and Research, Food and Drug Administration, Statement to Subcommittee on National Security, Veterans Affairs, and International Relations, 21 July 1999; on-line, internet, 19 February 2000, available from http://www.hhs.gov/progorg/asl/testify/t990721b.html.

77. Friedlander, "Anthrax Vaccine: Evidence for Safety and Efficacy Against Inhalation Anthrax," op. cit., 2104.

78. "Anthrax Vaccine – Safety."(no date); on-line, internet, 11 February 2000, available from http://www.anthrax.osd.mil/oldavip/qna/SAFETY.HTM.

79. "Anthrax Vaccine Adsorbed," Food and Drug Administration Required Product Insert; on-line, internet, 11 February 2000, available from http://bioportcorp.com/AnthraxIns.htm. See also, Myers, n.p.

80. Phillip S. Brachman, "Inhalation Anthrax," a public domain document originally published in *Annals of the New York Academy of Sciences,* 353, no date, 83-93.

81. F. Marc LaForce, "Anthrax," *Clinical Infectious Diseases,* 19 December 1994, 1009-1014. See also, "Vaccine Safety," no date; on-line, internet, 4 September 2000, available from http://www.anthrax.osd.mil/Site_Files/safety/safety_info.htm. See also, Hedlund, op. cit., 72-73.

82. *Federal Register.* See also, Lew, op. cit., 1886. See also, LaForce, op. cit., 1010.

83. Friedlander, "Anthrax Vaccine: Evidence for Safety and Efficacy Against Inhalation Anthrax," op. cit., 2105-2106.

84. The Food and Drug Administration has not approved Anthrax Vaccine, Adsorbed for use to protect against inhalation anthrax. But, lack of Food and Drug Administration approval for a specific indication does not prohibit the use of a medication for that indication if clinical evidence exists to support it. Food and Drug Administration licensure means that the medical product may be sold commercially in the U.S. Food and Drug Administration approval means testing for that indication has been completed according to Food and Drug Administration specifications in connection with the licensing process. Lack of Food and Drug Administration approval only means that the rigorous testing required by the Food and Drug Administration (paid for by the manufacturer) before it will grant its endorsement has not been completed. If there is reasonable clinical evidence to support using a medication for an indication not approved by the Food and Drug Administration, a physician may prescribe that medication for that use based on the physician's clinical judgment. Such use is also not considered experimental since the medication is already licensed. In a letter to the Honorable Dan Burton dated 26 November 1999, Melinda K. Plaisier, the Associate Commissioner for Legislation for the Food and Drug Administration, discusses the procedures by which lots are released by the Food and Drug Administration for sale and distribution. Regarding indications for use, she states, "The labeling for Anthrax Vaccine Adsorbed does not mention route of exposure (e.g., cutaneous) per se. Use of the vaccine for protection against both cutaneous and inhalation anthrax exposure is not inconsistent with the labeling for Anthrax Vaccine Adsorbed." She adds that there is no reason for Anthrax Vaccine, Adsorbed to be returned to an investigational new drug status when used to vaccinate against inhalation anthrax, especially since the rarity and risk of human inhalation anthrax precludes gathering additional clinical data.

85. Myers, op. cit. See also, "Medical Readiness: Issues Concerning the Anthrax Vaccine," Government Accounting Office Testimony before the Subcommittee on National Security, Veterans Affairs, and International Relations, 21 July 1999, Government Accounting Office /T-NSIAD-99-226, 7-9.

86. "Anthrax Vaccine Adsorbed," Food and Drug Administration Required Product Insert.

87. "Anthrax Vaccine – Safety," on-line, internet, 11 February 2000, available from http://www.anthrax.osd.mil/oldavip/qna/SAFETY.HTM.

88. Agency Group 09, "Surgeon General Testifies on Anthrax Vaccine," *FDCH Regulatory Intelligence Database,* 3 November 1999.

89. Friedlander, "Anthrax Vaccine: Evidence for Safety and Efficacy Against Inhalation Anthrax," 2104. See also, "Anthrax Vaccine Adsorbed," Food and Drug Administration Required Product Insert.

90. Ibid.

91. Ellenberg, op. cit.

92. *Federal Register*, op. cit.

93. "Anthrax Vaccine -- Safety," op. cit. See also, Mazzuchi, et al, op. cit., 261.

94. Friedlander, op. cit., 2105. See also, Mazzuchi, et al, op. cit., 261.

95. Ibid.

96. "Medical Readiness: Safety and Efficacy of the Anthrax Vaccine," Government Accounting Office Testimony before The Subcommittee on National Security, Veterans Affairs, and International Relations, 29 April 1999, GAO/T-NSIAD-99-148, 4-5.

97. Ibid., 4.

98. "Anaphylaxis in Relation to Anthrax Vaccination: Analysis by Anthrax Vaccine Immunization Program Agency," (2 December 1999), n.p.: on-line, internet, 12 August 2000, available from http://www.anthrax.osd.mil/SCANNED/ARTICLES/grabedocs/anaphylaxis.htm.

99. Inglesby, op. cit., 1735-1736, 1740, 1744.

100. "Anthrax Vaccine -- Safety," op. cit.

101. "Form, Vaccine Adverse Events Reporting System-1 Reports," 23 August 2000; on-line, internet, 26 August 2000, available from http://www.anthrax.osd.mil/HTML_interface/ \default.html.

102. Friedlander, "Anthrax Vaccine: Evidence for Safety and Efficacy Against Inhalation Anthrax," op. cit., 2105.

103. "Surveillance for Adverse Events Associated with Anthrax Vaccination – U.S. Department of Defense, 1998-2000, " *Morbidity and Mortality Weekly Report* 49, No. 16, 28 April 2000, 341-345; on-line, internet, 12 August 2000, available from http://www.cdc.gov/epo/mmwr/preview/mmwrhtml/mm4916a1.htm.

104. "Safety Review of Anthrax Vaccine, 24 April 2000," n.p.: on-line, Internet, 12 August 2000, available from http://www.anthrax.osd.mil/SCANNED/ARTICLES/grabedocs/safetyReview-Anthrax Vaccine, Adsorbed.htm.

105. Charles L. Cragin, Acting Secretary of Defense for Reserve Affairs, "The Anthrax Vaccine: Safe, Effective, and Necessary," *Defense Link*, August 1999; on-line, internet 11 February 2000, available from http://www.defenselink.mil/news/Aug1999?n08171999_9908176.html. See also Myers, op. cit.

106. Friedlander, "Anthrax Vaccine: Evidence for Safety and Efficacy Against Inhalation Anthrax," op. cit., 2105.

107. "Safety Review of Anthrax Vaccine, 24 April 2000," op. cit.

108. Myers, op. cit.

109. Friedlander, "Anthrax Vaccine: Evidence for Safety and Efficacy Against Inhalation Anthrax," 2104, 2106.

110. Jamie McIntyre, "All U.S. Troops to get Anthrax Vaccine," *CNN Interactive,* 15 December 1997; on-line, internet, 17 February 2000, available from http://cnn.com?U.S./9712/15/military.anthrax/. See also, Cragin, op. cit., and Mazzuchi, et al., op. cit., 261.

111. Inglesby, op. cit., 1735. See also, *MMWR,* 28 April 2000, and Friedlander, "Anthrax Vaccine: Evidence for Safety and Efficacy Against Inhalation Anthrax," op. cit., 2104.

112. Peter Bergen, et al., "Terror Network Eyeing U.S. Outposts Worldwide, Officials Say," *CNN,* 17 June 1999; on-line, internet, 17 February 2000, available from http://cnn.com/U.S./9906/17/bin.laden.threat/.

113. David Ensor, "Panel: U.S. Not Prepared to Combat Weapons of Mass Destruction," *CNN,* 8 July 1999; on-line, internet, 17 February 2000, available from http://cnn.com/U.S./9907/08/us.threat.study/.

114. House, *A Bill to suspend further implementation of the Department of Defense Anthrax Vaccination Program until the vaccine is determined to be safe and effective and to provide for a full study by the National Institutes of Health of that vaccine,* 106th Cong., 1st session, 1999, H.R. 2548; on-line, internet, 14 February 2000, available from http://www.dallasnw.quik.com/cyberella/Anthrax/HR_2548.html.

115. Hedlund, op. cit., 48.

116. Laura Laughlin, "Shot to Hell," *Phoenixnewtimes.com,* 27 January 2000; on-line, internet, 14 February 2000, available from http://www.phoenixnewtimes.com/issues/2000-01-27/feature.html.

117. Clement, op. cit., 70-71.

118. Al Hinman, "Scientists: U.S. Must Prepare for Biological Warfare," *CNN Interactive,* 11 March 1998; on-line, internet, 17 February 2000, available from http://cnn.com/HEALTH/9803/11/bioterrorism/index.html.

119. Clement, op. cit., 93.

120. Hedlund, op. cit., 76.

121. "Anthrax Vaccine Links and Information," on-line, internet, 27 August 2000, available from http://www.dallasnw.quik.com/cyberella/index.htm.

122. Thomas L. Rempfer, "Why Am I Resisting the Vaccine? The Military Trained Me To," *Washingtonpost.com,* 30 January, 2000; on-line, internet, 5 February 2000, available from http://www.washingtonpost.com/wp-srv/Wplate/2000-01/30/1531-013000-idx.html. See also, "Anthrax Vaccine Protestors Gather Outside Air Force Base," *Miami Herald,* 29 January 2000; on-line, internet, 5 February 2000, available from http://www.herald.com/content/today/digdocs/026528.htm.

123. Lieutenant General (retired) James Terry Scott, "In Defending Its Troop Against Anthrax, The Pentagon Has Injected Distrust Instead," *Washingtonpost.com,* 30 January 2000; on-line, internet, 5 February 2000, available from http://www.washingtonpost.com/wp-srv/Wplate/2000-01-30-1511-013000.idx.html.

124. "Anthrax Vaccine Immunization Program," (no date); on-line, internet, 11 February 2000, available from http://www.anthrax.osd.mil/.

125. Kathryn C. Zoon, letter, 28 April 1998; on-line, internet, 4 September 2000, available from http://www.dallasnw.quik.com/cyberella/Anthrax/Zoon4_98.html.

126. John Davidson, "Anti bio-weapon vaccine for troops fails safety tests," *Independent,* 6 December 1999; on-line, internet, 2 September 2000, available from http://www.dallasnw.quik.com/cyberella/Anthrax/UKHealth.html.

127. Ibid.

128. Several independent nationally renowned scientific groups have addressed this issue and have found no evidence to link anthrax vaccine with illnesses among Gulf War veterans. There have been several unsubstantiated allegations in the media and elsewhere about experimental vaccines that may have contained non-Food and Drug Administration-licensed substances such as squalene. Only the Food and Drug Administration-licensed anthrax vaccines have been used. See "Anthrax Vaccine and the Persian Gulf War," on-line, internet, 15 February 2000, available at http://www.anthrax.osd.mil/oldavip/qna/GULFWAR.HTM.)

129. "Anthrax Vaccine Links and Information," op. cit.

130. "Memorandum of Understanding Between the Food and Drug Administration and the Department of Defense Concerning Investigational Use of Drugs, Antibiotics, and Medical Devices by the Department of Defense," 1 May 1987; on-line, internet, 4 September 2000, available from http://www.dallasnw.quik.com/cyberella/Anthrax/MOU.html.

131. Laughlin, op. cit.

132. "Food and Drug Administration Inspection Cites Problems in Anthrax Vaccine Production," *Associated Press,* 15 December 1999; on-line, internet, 14 February 2000, available from http.../AppLogic+FTContentServer?section=archieve&pagename= story&storyid=115019020857.

133. "Anthrax Vaccine Links and Information."

134. Those opposed to the use of Anthrax Vaccine, Adsorbed and the Anthrax Vaccine Immunization Program are likely to point out that the Defense Department information web sites, promoting the safety and efficacy of Anthrax Vaccine, Adsorbed, are also biased. The influence of bias in any presentation of opinion regarding Anthrax Vaccine, Adsorbed and the Anthrax Vaccine Immunization Program makes it even more essential to base decisions regarding vaccination policy on documented facts.

135. Laughlin, op. cit.

136. "Anthrax Vaccine Home Page," (no date), n.p.; on-line, internet, 11 February 2000, available at http://www.anthraxvaccine.org/.

137. "Dr. Meryl Nass," (no date), n.p.; on-line, internet, 27 August 2000, available at http://www.dallasnw.quik.com/cyberella/Anthrax/credentials.html.

138. Laughlin.

139. Nass, "Anthrax Vaccine," 187-208.

140. Ibid., 199.

141. Ibid., 203.

142. Meryl Nass, "Ádverse Effects: Anthrax Vaccine," on-line, internet, 27 August 2000, available from http://www.anthraxvaccine.org/adveffcts.htm.

143. "Medical Readiness: Safety and Efficacy of the Anthrax Vaccine," op. cit., 3-4.

144. It is important to remember that General Accounting Office (GAO) testimonies are intended to present the results of fact-finding inquiries. Those conducting the investigations for the GAO may not be experts in the topic being investigated. The GAO official giving testimony appears before Congress to enter the facts resulting from the investigation into the record without any editorializing, comments, or conclusions. As in any legal proceeding, the facts entered during the GAO testimony may not be all the facts. The GAO testimonies should be balanced and cross-examined with additional facts

and testimony from witnesses and experts before any decisions or conclusions are reached. The "Anthrax Vaccine Links and Information" site and Dr. Nass tend to take portions of GAO testimony and draw conclusions without considering statements entered into the Congressional record by other witnesses, placing facts entered during GAO testimonies into context.

145. Nass, "Ádverse Effects: Anthrax Vaccine," op. cit.

146. Ellenberg, op. cit.

147. Gina Terracciano, Robert Chen, Jenifer Lloyd, "Surveillance for Adverse Events Following Vaccination," September 1997; on-line, Internet, 15 February 2000, available from http://www.cdc.gov/nip/vacsafe/vaccinesafety/publications/aesurveillance.htm.

148. Ellenberg, op. cit.

149. Nass, "Ádverse Effects: Anthrax Vaccine," op. cit.

150. Friedlander, "Anthrax Vaccine: Evidence for Safety and Efficacy Against Inhalation Anthrax," op. cit., 2105.

151. Lieutenant General Hal M. Hornberg, "Vaccine is Safe, Effective," *Air Force Times,* 60, Issue 16, 22 November 1999, 55.

152. Anthrax Vaccine, Adsorbed has been administered to thousands of veterinary and laboratory workers, livestock handlers since 1970. In addition, there have been at least four major independent reviews by civilian panels on the safety and efficacy of Anthrax Vaccine, Adsorbed. See "Vaccine Safety," no-date, on-line, internet, 4 September 2000, available from http://www.anthrax.osd.mil/Site_Files/safety/safety_info.htm.

153. It should be noted that the strength of clinical evidence would be enhanced if more data were published in the peer-reviewed literature, and researchers should be encouraged to submit their data to the peer-review process. ("An Assessment of the Safety of the Anthrax Vaccine: A Letter Report.")

154. Ibid.

155. Nass, "Anthrax Vaccine," op. cit., 203. See also, Nass, "Anthrax Vaccine Safety and Efficacy: Response to the Army Surgeon General Ronald Blanck's Posting," op. cit.

156. Ken Alibek, *Biohazard,* (New York, NY: Random House, 1999), 261,281. See also, Inglesby, op. cit., 1744.

157. Dr. Nass cites a study in which different strains of anthrax were tested in guinea pigs vaccinated with Anthrax Vaccine, Adsorbed. In the study, 9 of 27 strains appeared to be resistant to vaccination. See Nass, "Anthrax Vaccine Safety and Efficacy: Response to the Army Surgeon General Ronald Blanck's Posting," op. cit. Friedlander, "Anthrax Vaccine: Evidence for Safety and Efficacy Against Inhalation Anthrax,"

however, provides a thorough review of several animal studies, including the study cited by Dr. Nass, in which Anthrax Vaccine, Adsorbed is tested against various strains of anthrax in several different animal species. He demonstrates that, while Anthrax Vaccine, Adsorbed provided variable protection against certain strains of anthrax in guinea pigs, Anthrax Vaccine, Adsorbed provided excellent protection against even the most virulent and seemingly resistant strains (such as the Ames strain) in non-human primates and rabbits, even after just two doses of the vaccine. This most likely reflects species-specific differences with the guinea pig's immune system, making it more difficult to immunize the guinea pig against anthrax compared to other animal species, and is not due to any strain of anthrax developing resistance to the anthrax vaccine. (Friedlander, "Anthrax Vaccine: Evidence for Safety and Efficacy Against Inhalation Anthrax," op. cit., 2105-2106.)

158. Nass, "Anthrax Vaccine," op. cit., 189. See also, Inglesby, op. cit., 1744.

159. New anthrax vaccines have been developed and are ready for clinical testing. But so far, lack of funding has prevented the performance of clinical trial studies. (LaForce, op. cit., 1013.)

160. Laughlin, op. cit.

161. Ibid., 1735. See also, Clement, op. cit., 53-54, 79.

162. Nass, "Anthrax Vaccine," op. cit., 204. See also, Inglesby, op. cit., 1735.

163. Havrilak, op. cit.

164. Hedlund, op. cit., 76.

165. "Anthrax Vaccine Casualties at One Military Installation," no date; on-line, internet, 2 September 2000, available from http://www.dallasnw.quik.com/cyberella/Anthrax/dover4-1.html.

166. Friedlander, "Anthrax Vaccine: Evidence for Safety and Efficacy Against Inhalation Anthrax," op. cit., 2104.

167. Dr. Nass reports the results of a survey sent out to members of the 9th Airlift Squadron at Dover Air Force Base. In this report, she admits that the survey results cannot be used to establish that Anthrax Vaccine, Adsorbed actually caused the symptoms due to the lack of a control group. Overall, 252 surveys were sent out, and 139 were completed and returned. She interprets 81 as probably having a systemic reaction due to Anthrax Vaccine, Adsorbed. At least six indicated they felt Anthrax Vaccine, Adsorbed did not cause their symptoms. Even though she admits there can be no statistical analysis of this data and it is not possible to prove causality, Dr. Nass concludes something must be wrong at Dover because it is just not normal for so many otherwise healthy people at one location to be having symptoms or strange illnesses of one sort or another. A useful analysis would be to compare the rate of occurrence of symptoms and diseases in 9th Airlift Squadron personnel against the rate of occurrence in

all unvaccinated personnel at Dover and the U.S. population in general, but this is not provided. Nor is there an attempt to look for recurring patterns of symptoms. Indeed, it appears from the survey results that the patterns of symptoms vary widely, with no two individuals' symptom patterns matching. (Meryl Nass, "Survey Results of the 9th Airlift Squadron," op. cit., no date; on-line, internet, 27 August 2000, available from http://www.anthraxvaccine.org.)

168. Lieutenant General Paul K. Carlton, Jr., "Anthrax," no date; on-line, internet, 4 September 2000, available from http://sg-www.satx.disa.mil/af/sg/presentations/Anthrax_Threat.ppt.

169. H.R.2548. See also, Mike Ahlers, "Congressional Panel Recommends Suspension of Military's Anthrax Vaccine," *CNN,* 17 February 2000; on-line, internet, 17 February 2000, available from http://cnn.com.

170. Scott, op. cit.

171. Ibid.

172. Ibid.

173. "An Assessment of the Safety of the Anthrax Vaccine: A Letter Report," op cit.

174. The letter, dated 30 March 2000, is the result of a request the Secretary of Defense sent to the Institute of Medicine to assess the safety of Anthrax Vaccine, Adsorbed. The Institute of Medicine commented that its assessment is an early step in sorting out the complex issues surrounding Anthrax Vaccine, Adsorbed and has started a two-year in-depth study that will include a review of all available data from the Department of Defense. ("A Letter Report from the Institute of Medicine (IOM), 30 March 2000," no date; on-line, internet, 12 August 2000, available from http://www.anthrax.osd.mil/SCANNED/ARTICLES/ltrReportINtro.htm.)

175. Inglesby, op. cit., 1740.

www.ingramcontent.com/pod-product-compliance
Lightning Source LLC
Chambersburg PA
CBHW081258180526
45170CB00007B/2479